Contents

The Lavender Trust Fund

The Lavender Trust was set up in memory of the journalist Ruth Picardie by the late Beth Wagstaff in order to develop further the unique range of services that the national charity Breast Cancer Care offers to younger women with breast cancer, their partners and families. In total, 33 000 women (and 200 men) are diagnosed with breast cancer each year in the UK. Of these, 20% of the women are premenopausal, and as well as facing concerns that are common to all women, there are often unique issues which younger women may also face.

Already enough money has been raised to:

- recruit a younger women's specialist nurse
- extend the helpline opening hours to include Saturday from June 2000
- produce booklets and factsheets
- launch a website at www.lavendertrustfund.org.uk which provides details of the charity's unique services for younger women, as well as the opportunity to order free literature on a wide range of breast cancer concerns
- hold telephone support groups throughout the year
- recruit and train younger women volunteers.

For further information, contact the Lavender Trust on 020 7384 4617 or email ltf@breastcancercare.org.uk, or visit the website.

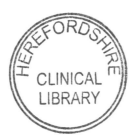

Conference of Postgraduate Advisers in General Practice, Universities of the UK

UKCRA is an independent national forum of discussion and action on all matters related to education and training for general practice. Its aims and objectives are to be concerned with all matters relating to general practice education and training, including the following.

1   Contribution to the formulation of national and regional policies.
2   Responding constructively to the decisions made by other national organisations.
3   Providing a useful forum for exchange of information and relevant data.
4   Providing stimulus for change and improvement in quality.
5   Participating actively in national debates by seeking and maintaining representation on the various national organisations.
6   Promoting and providing appropriate educational activities for its members.
7   Disseminating relevant information and data to all its constituents.
8   Identifying and promoting relevant research and appropriate development.
9   Continuing to liaise with the relevant UK organisations and institutions.
10 Providing advice and guidance on accreditation of distance-based learning programmes and overseas meetings.
11 Advising on the career structure and development for course organisers, associate advisers, GP tutors, directors of postgraduate GP education and trainers.
12 Encouraging and undertaking audit and performance review when appropriate.

UKCRA has achieved much over recent years:

- the drafting of the first constitution of the conference
- establishing National Accreditation Panels for distance-based learning programmes and international courses
- the inclusion of associate advisers/deputies as full members of the UK Conference
- discussing and defining the role of the regional advisers, and their terms and conditions of service

- addressing the educational needs of the advisers and deputies by running annual residential educational meetings, hosted by different deaneries in rotation
- setting up the UK Conference Working Panels on Summative Assessment
- implementing the Joint Committee policy in establishing a clear procedure for Summative Assessment.

Dr Simon Smail is the Chairman of UKCRA and Dr Neil Jackson, the Secretary.

Preface

Doctors have been thrust into the spotlight by the Bristol, Shipman and Ledward scandals. The profession has not helped itself by tearing itself apart over the role of the General Medical Council and the nature of the future revalidation process. The Government has sensed the public's concern and set a challenge that could be perceived as threatening to the way in which general practice has traditionally operated. However, it can also be viewed as presenting us with opportunities. Choice is not an option – we have to assimilate the changes, we must rise to the challenges, demonstrate leadership and become the architects of change, rather than be the passive recipients of edicts from elsewhere.

This book aims to provide inspiration to its readers and fuel for the challenges ahead. It is an anthology of work produced by many of the leading figures in general practice across the UK. It started life in the summer of 2000 at the UKCRA annual conference held at Warwick University. The theme of the conference was the 'General Practice Jigsaw'. It proved to be highly enjoyable and successful. Many people suggested that the workshops and presentations should be further developed to offer this book as the most up-to-date resource available.

The purpose of the book is to share knowledge and best practice with regard to general practice education, teaching and professional development, drawing on examples from across the UK, including local, regional and national projects. The book is aimed not only at general practitioners involved in education and training, but also at all members of primary healthcare teams who want to be involved in shaping the primary care organisations of the future.

Steve Field
Bob Strachan
Gai Evans
February 2001

About the editors

Steve Field is director of postgraduate general practice education for the West Midlands, vice-chair of the Committee of GP Education Directors (COGPED) and chair of the Implementation Committee for the new UK GP Registrar Scheme. He has been a GP since 1986, and is a GP principal in inner-city Birmingham. He is an MRCGP examiner and a member of the RCGP's examination board. He is convinced that poor communication skills lead to poor outcomes for patients, and he is therefore committed to developing and supporting the teaching, learning and assessment of communication skills in general practice.

Bob Strachan is associate director for Birmingham and Solihull in the West Midlands. He has been a GP since 1969 in a long-established training practice teaching both GP registrars and undergraduate medical students. He was a course organiser for six years, and has organised the Warwick GP Trainers' Courses for many years. He has pioneered the use of practice managers as part of the accreditation of training practices, and has played an active part in the development of multiprofessional education in the region. He chaired the organising committee of the UKCRA conference in June 2000.

Gai Evans has worked for the West Midlands Postgraduate GP Education Unit for three years as personal assistant to Steve Field, and more recently as recruitment officer for the West Midlands following the introduction of the new enhanced management arrangements for vocational training. She was responsible for the organisation and administration of the successful 'General Practice Jigsaw' UKCRA Conference at Warwick University in June 2000.

List of contributors

Nafsika Alexiadou, Education Department, Keele University

Justin Allen, Joint Honorary Secretary, Joint Committee on Postgraduate Training for General Practice (JCPTGP), London, and Deputy Director of Postgraduate General Practice Education, South Trent Deanery

Margareth Attwood, GP Project Manager, Wessex Deanery

Jamie Bahrami, Director of Postgraduate General Practice Education, Yorkshire Deanery

Reed Bowden, Associate Dean (Assessment), North Thames (East) Deanery

Terry Bradley, Associate Director of General Practice Education, Northern Ireland

Laurence Buckman, Member of the BMA General Practitioners' Committee and Member of the RCGP Revalidation Working Group and the Good Medical Practice Working Party

Ruth Chambers, Professor of Primary Care Development, School of Health, Staffordshire University

Maureen Crawford, Associate Director of General Practice Education, Northern Ireland

Phil Croft, Senior Role-Player, Department of Primary Care and General Practice, University of Birmingham

Paul Downey, Course Organiser, Hereford Vocational Training Scheme

Alison Evans, Research and Development Fellow, Yorkshire Deanery

Steve Field, Director of Postgraduate General Practice Education, West Midlands NHS Executive, and Chair, MRCGP and Summative Assessment Liaison Group

Michael Fisher, Associate Director, West Midlands Deanery

Michael Greco, Deputy Director, Audit and Information Management Technology

Nicholas Greenfield, Director, Birmingham and Solihull Education Consortium

Mike Grenville, Associate Dean, North Thames (East)

Christopher Hand, Associate Adviser for General Practice Postgraduate Education, East Anglia Deanery, and Honorary Senior Lecturer, School of Health Policy and Practice, University of East Anglia, Norwich

Alexander Heazell, Pre-Registration House Officer, Dudley, West Midlands

Arthur Hibble, Director of Postgraduate General Practice Education, East Anglia Deanery

John Holden, General Practitioner Trainer and Member of RCGP Membership by Assessment of Performance Implementation Group

Guy Houghton, Associate Director (West Midlands) and Clinical Director, Birmingham Health Authority Clinical Governance Support Unit

Neil Jackson, Director of Postgraduate General Practice Education, North Thames (East) Deanery

Andrew Kelly, Pre-Registration House Officer, Coventry rotation 1998

Diane Kelly, Assistant Director for Continuing Professional Development, West of Scotland

Stephen Kelly, Deputy Director of Postgraduate General Practice Education, West Midlands Region

Pat Lane, Director of Postgraduate General Practice Education, North Trent Region

Murray Lough, Assistant Director, Audit and Information Management Technology, West of Scotland

Ian McLean, Associate Adviser, South Thames East Deanery

Monica McLean, Department of Education, University of Keele

Anne McKee, Educational Research Fellow for General Practice Post-graduate Education, East Anglia Deanery, and Senior Research Associate, Centre for Applied Research in Education (CARE), School of Education and Professional Development, University of East Anglia, Norwich

Janet Marjoram, Practice Manager, Hawthorns Surgery, Sutton Coldfield

Katharine Messenger, Senior Role-Player, Department of Primary Care and General Practice, University of Birmingham

Lesley Millard, Education Adviser, South Thames East, Department of Postgraduate General Practice Education

Bitty Muller, Associate Adviser for GP Non-Principals, West Midlands Region

Philip Nolan, Deputy Director of Postgraduate General Practice Education

Dec O'Brien, Course Organiser, Hereford Vocational Training Scheme

Fiona Patterson, Lecturer, Department of Occupational Psychology, University of Sheffield

Ed Peile, NHS Fellow, Oxford

John Pitts, Associate Director of Postgraduate General Practice Education, Wessex Deanery

Mike Pringle, Chairman of Council, Royal College of General Practitioners

Claire Rayner, Chairperson, Patients' Association

Trefor Roscoe, GP Informatics Tutor, North Trent, and Honorary Lecturer, Institute of General Practice, University of Sheffield Medical School

John Skelton, Senior Lecturer and Director, Interactive Skills Unit, Department of Primary Care and General Practice, University of Birmingham

Simon Smail, Sub-Dean and Director, Department of Postgraudate Education for General Practice, University of Wales College of Medicine, Cardiff

David Snadden, Director of Postgraduate General Practice Education, Dundee

Bob Strachan, Associate Director, Birmingham and Solihull, West Midlands Region

Malcolm Valentine, Associate Regional Adviser, North-East Scotland, and Vice-Chairman of the National Association of GP Tutors

Rebecca Viney, Primary Care Tutor and Course Organiser for GP Non-Principals, North Thames (East) Deanery

Gill Wakley, Clinical Governance Tutor, School of Health, Staffordshire University

David Wall, General Practitioner, Sutton Coldfield, and Acting Regional Postgraduate Dean, University of Birmingham and West Midlands Deanery

Robin While, Associate Director, Wessex Deanery

Connie Wiskin, Co-ordinator for Interactive Teaching, Department of Primary Care and General Practice, University of Birmingham

Acknowledgements

The UKCRA Conference 2000 took over a year to plan, and was the product of excellent teamwork within the West Midlands Postgraduate General Practice Education Unit. It proved to be a great success. The chairman of the organising committee was Bob Strachan, who worked way beyond the call of duty. The person who pulled everything together and organised the speakers, workshops and accommodation was Gai Evans, who also helped to edit this book. Dean Bruton, the office manager, was invaluable, as was my tireless deputy, Stephen Kelly. Carol Harper, Barbara Lloyd, Fiona Kavanagh, Sharon Robinson and Beryl Smith were also extremely helpful and supportive. A big thank you to you all!

Because of the importance of the subjects presented and discussed in the workshops, many participants said that they thought that the proceedings should be made more widely available. Gillian Nineham of Radcliffe Medical Press attended the conference and encouraged us to expand on the presentations and develop them into a book. We are therefore indebted to Gillian, who has seen this project through to completion.

Lynn Field had a key role in keeping me sane while I was bringing the different strands of the book together, by rewriting the occasional paragraph and checking that my English was up to date! Janet Marjoram has also contributed significantly to the development of the book. Thank you both once again! We promise that we shall not suggest that we host another national conference for many years!

Steve Field
February 2001

List of abbreviations

CME	Continuing medical education
CMO	Chief Medical Officer
COGPED	Committee of General Practice Education Directors
COPMeD	Committee of Postgraduate Medical Deans
CPD	Continuing professional development
DPGPE	Director of Postgraduate General Practice Education
FRCGP	Fellow of the Royal College of General Practitioners
GMC	General Medical Council
GMS	General Medical Services (those services provided by general practitioners)
GP	General practitioner
GPASS	General Practitioner Administrative System for Scotland
JCPTGP	Joint Committee on Postgraduate Training for General Practice
LMC	Local Medical Committee
MAAG	Medical Audit Advisory Group
MADEL	Medical and Dental Education Levy
MRCGP	Member of the Royal College of General Practitioners
MRCP	Member of the Royal College of Physicians
NSF	National service framework
OSCE	objective structured clinical examination
PAM	profession allied to medicine
PCG	Primary care group
PCT	Primary care trust
PDP	Personal development plan
PMS	Personal medical services
PPDP	Practice and professional development plan
PRHO	Pre-registration house officer
RCGP	Royal College of General Practitioners
SHO	Senior house officer
SpR	Specialist registrar
UCAS	University and Colleges Admission Service
UKCRA	United Kingdom Conference of Regional Advisers
VTS	Vocational training scheme

Working together

Mike Pringle

Professor Mike Pringle was invited to the UKCRA conference to give a short presentation on the future of general practice education and training.

He discussed five key areas.

Training for general practice

He argued that the 1979 'deal' – revolutionary and remarkable in its time – was now ready for review and renewal. He emphasised the need to select GP registrars who have appropriate human and scientific attributes to become effective general practitioners. He reinforced the need for training to be targeted on the skills and attributes of a new general practitioner. He added that we should continue to campaign for the length of GP training to be flexible in order to meet the needs of the registrar (as it is for hospital registrars). He also supported the call for GP registrars to be able to undertake as much of the training as is appropriate in general practice settings.

Entry into general practice

He argued for the MRCGP examination to become compulsory for future GP principals in general practice. He acknowledged that summative assessment was a considerable advance on the old 'certificate of satisfactory completion', and added that he believed that it is not acceptable that doctors should continue to enter general practice with such a low-standard qualification.

The early years

The case for higher professional education (HPE) through the early years was made. Professor Pringle called for preparation for a lifetime in general practice, which includes effective vocational training and then further support during the doctor's working career. He said that this must include training in team-working, research, commissioning, ethics, practice management, etc. – all skills that are best acquired when facing real issues. New doctors need mentoring and support in establishing the habit of lifelong learning, he said, and personal medical services (PMS) offers new flexibility in contracts. However, he cautioned that we have a responsibility to ensure that young doctors are not exploited.

Inspiring quality of care

Professor Pringle went on to outline the attributes of a GP that should be encouraged, namely reflection, lifelong learning, communication skills, professional values and clinical performance. He continued by listing some mechanisms that can be used to instil and develop these attributes. These include significant event auditing, conventional auditing, continuing professional development (CPD), clinical governance, responding to complaints and suggestions, and listening to patients.

While there are personal or team issues, there are also external imperatives. Professor Pringle called for the profession to accept some responsibility for addressing issues such as rationing, evidence-based care, and the implementation of national service frameworks (NSFs) and National Institute for Clinical Excellence (NICE) guidelines. In addition, he said that there is a responsibility to define the value and benefits of and to aspire to live up to the promise of generalism, as a key component of the healthcare system.

Demonstrating quality

Professor Pringle outlined methods for assessing quality in individual GPs. These included revalidation, accredited professional development, membership by assessment of performance, fellowship by assessment, trainer recognition and higher degrees. He then looked at quality markers for teams, including quality team development, quality practice award, training practice approval and accreditation for R&D in general practice.

Working together

Professor Pringle concluded by looking at how this vision could be achieved. It clearly requires the College and the educationalists to work together. Only through close co-operation can we hope to deliver on such a complex and demanding agenda.

Part 1

The patient's perspective

There have been considerable changes in primary care since the introduction of the 'new contract' in 1990, but there seems to have been little change in the factors that patients consider important and which demonstrate high-quality care.

Miss Rayner, Chairperson of the Patients' Association, reminds us of the importance of the doctor–patient relationship, empathy and understanding, and the receiving and giving of information to an increasingly well-informed patient. She emphasises that patients need to have trust and confidence in their doctor. This is particularly important in the present climate of publicity given to medical mistakes. Miss Rayner's comments support the principle that consultation skills training needs to continue to form a significant part of the curriculum of vocational training for general practitioners. Doctors will increasingly need to demonstrate the quality and effectiveness of this inter-action within the privacy of their surgery.

In the following chapter, Michael Greco builds on some of the issues raised by Miss Rayner and introduces the Doctors' Interpersonal Skills Questionnaire (DISQ), which has been designed to give general practitioners structured feedback on their interpersonal skills within the consultation. DISQ could well become a tool that is used to provide evidence for revalidation purposes – a hot topic!

1

The patient's perspective

Claire Rayner

> My own understanding of the NHS started when I trained as a midwife in the days when 60% of mothers were delivered in hospital and 40% had home deliveries but it was thought you weren't really a midwife until you had a baby yourself. To have had a general anaesthetic yourself gives you a much better notion of what a patient faces and might be feeling. You get even more frightened than the patient of course because you really know what can go wrong, but patients also have a pretty good idea.
>
> Claire Rayner, Chairperson of the Patients' Association

The doctor–patient relationship

The notion that patients are seen as passive recipients of what is available and what is offered, and that they are there to have things done *to* them and *for* them is now outdated. We have undergone a massive change, and many patients are now fairly well informed.

Some older patients may prefer to be helpless and passive, although most are informed and to an extent 'consumerised' – people whom you do things not to and for, but *with*. This changes the doctor–patient relationship profoundly. The 'informed' patients are not the people to whom experts and professionals can apply their knowledge. Patients regard doctors as 'expert guides' on the road for which they already have a map, even though for some it may be a very rudimentary map and for others a detailed one.

The Patients' Association was born in the middle of a consumerist revolution in the 1960s. It was very confrontational, very abrasive, very anti-doctor for a very long time. Now it is more of a consensual organisation, pushing the fact that patients are a resource, too. The Patients' Association exerts pressure for change, offers constructive ideas for improvement in the service, and generally runs around biting the rear ends of those in power. It gains much of its information from its helpline. People telephone The Patients' Association for all sorts of reasons, and for all sorts of information.

Quality of care

What does quality mean? And what does it mean to a patient? Patients do not think of the NHS as segmented into primary, secondary and tertiary care, but rather they imagine it as a seamless service. An important point to remember is that what matters to patients about an episode of ill health is not the individual components, but rather the total experience of the NHS. Thus a mother may go to hospital and be given superb quality of care through a difficult delivery, but she may then complain about the quality of the food and the fact that it was noisy at night. People may think 'ungrateful cow', but this is not the case – she is doing what I think most of us would do in her situation, looking at the total experience. She is unaware of how much expertise went into her delivery – all she knows is that she was not properly fed.

Patients need to feel complete trust both in the people who care for them and for their relatives, and in the system within which that care is provided. It is very important that they can trust the quality of doctor training. They also need to be sure that all of the people who do care for them have been properly trained and have also been well supervised at all levels. The GMC is important to them. Patients also need to know that medical staff are listed on a register which is used by employers and local authorities to ensure that all staff are eligible, properly qualified, properly trained and have nothing in their past to make them ineligible.

It is important that the staff who look after patients are provided with proper working conditions and remuneration. We know perfectly well that unhappy workers, however powerful their vocation for their work, cannot give of their best. Since it is their best that we most need when we are ill and vulnerable, the welfare of doctors, nurses and other staff is of concern to us, if only as a form of enlightened self-interest.

Empathy and understanding

Patients are desperately vulnerable. Anyone who has ever been ill will know how very exposed a patient feels. It is as if someone has peeled three skins off you and you do need a sense of safety – it is an almost child-like situation. I would remind you to bear in mind how vulnerable we are even if we are exuding self-confidence. In the experience of The Patients' Association it is very rare for any individual to speak to anyone – be they a doctor or a nurse – about anything to do with their own health without experiencing a certain amount of inner discomfort.

No reasonable patient would condone rudeness or violence towards hospital or practice workers, but I do think it is important to bear in mind that fear and anxiety have a profound effect on people. They rapidly create tension and aggression and, if pushed too far, violence. Next time you find yourself intervening in a scene between a receptionist or one of the practice staff and a patient, however irritable you may be and angered by the way in which the patient is behaving, it is extremely important to remember that he or she may have very valid reasons for behaving like this, even if you do not recognise them as such. Carers also come into this category. Sometimes you will find that a relative or a carer is much more aggressive, hostile and angry when they are acting on behalf of the patient. This can be very difficult to handle. The fear of loss of someone you love or the fear of damage or distress to your peaceful life and the threat to your own personal future can be very profound. Thus if a man becomes very aggressive when his wife comes in for treatment, it is not just a matter of him being a nasty soul – it could well be that he is going through the most appalling scenarios in his head, and perhaps he needs some information to reassure him. Losing one's temper with him will only make him worse. The Patients' Association receives many calls on the helpline about unpleasant attitudes displayed by healthcare workers and practice staff: 'they are short and crisp and have no time to talk, and that's what makes them ratty'. Many patients do admit to losing their tempers and being rude, and they want to know what they can do to put the matter right. The Patients' Association suggests that they should write a letter saying 'I'm very sorry I lost my temper, but this is why and how I was feeling'. We have received some very positive feedback from people who have used that method.

Informing the patient

Information is the most important general need: 'What is the matter with me?' 'Is it my fault, did I do it?' The first thing a mother may ask when her baby develops chicken-pox rash is 'What did I do, doctor? Where did I go wrong?' Just making patients feel less guilty can have an enormous beneficial effect. People want information about their condition – both general facts and support information. There is an enormous voluntary network outside the NHS, with an association for every illness under the sun. These associations produce extremely useful information leaflets. 'Start Here' is a touch screen system. You touch a button that says 'Help', and up comes a menu, under which there is a list of conditions. For example, if your patient has acne and they touch 'Acne', a list of possibilities will come up, including signs, symptoms, possible treatments, etc. There is a company that makes CD-ROMs which explain various conditions. Patients will benefit from this wide range of information, and an enormous amount of time will be saved in the long term. This is what is meant by being the expert guide and giving and improving rudimentary maps.

Efficiency of the service

There is nothing more frustrating than trying to phone a practice or a hospital department and getting one of those automatic 'if you have a touch-tone phone' lists. Not everyone has a touch-tone telephone, and they are also expensive for people on low incomes. It is important that people are able to telephone to cancel appointments, rather than being labelled a 'DNA' and scolded for not turning up and thus wasting NHS money. It is very frustrating and makes people very angry indeed.

Efficiency is not just about telephone systems. It is cruel to fail to let patients know the results of tests, so that they become frantically worried. I am thinking particularly of women who have had cervical smears and, when the result comes back to the practice, because of the system that is used it goes straight into the notes instead of to the practitioner, so no one bothers to tell the patient that she is clear. If there is an abnormal result you are more likely to be in touch with the patient. Other situations that cause endless problems and anxiety include the loss of samples in the pathology laboratory, labelling of samples with the wrong name, doing the wrong test or sending the results to the wrong person. Patients obviously feel very frightened when this happens. Being called to the surgery at short notice is another such situation, which upsets the practice as much as the patient.

The *total* experience is what matters to the patient. Patients cannot understand why *you* have not got the clout at the hospital. They think you ought to be able to say 'Why is this happening? Put it right'. It damages the relationship with you if you are unable to do so, so fight your hospitals even harder – this may seem a terrible thing to say, but I think in some cases you might have to.

Communication

If you decide that a patient is no longer persona gratis in your practice, then tell them why. If you strike them off, tell them why. If it is because they have an unpleasant, disagreeable or aggressive personality and no one can stand them, then tell them so. They are never going to improve if you do not. If they are over-demanding, may I suggest that you regard that as a sickness in itself.

Patients who are constantly attending – the hypochondriac, the malingerer, the over-anxious, the heart sinkers – are sick people. They are not making pests of themselves because they want to be a nuisance or because they just like coming to the surgery. Striking these patients off does not solve the problem – it just passes the problem on to someone else and frightens the patient even more.

The Patients' Association receives a large number of calls about patients being removed from their doctor's list, and many people telephone saying that they are very frightened that they will not continue to receive medical treatment, particularly if the drugs they need become too expensive. The recent fuss about beta-interferon has not helped. It does seem absurd that it has not been possible to devise some sort of system, for example, for testing people with multiple sclerosis to see what percentage respond to beta-interferon. Surely it ought to be possible, without spending a fortune, to undertake short test periods for a new drug, or an expensive one, in order to see who will bene-fit. I know that the prescribing of very costly medicines is out of your hands, but sometimes patients think that this is something you could help them with more than you do at present.

Patients need an honest and careful assessment of how much they should be involved in their own care. We are a difficult lot – on the one hand, 'tell us what's going on, answer our questions, give us all the information we want', and on the other, 'it's too much, we can't handle it, you make up your mind, you're the doctor'. There is a terribly difficult balance to be struck here. There again, we receive calls from women who say 'I've got this lump in my breast. My doctor says I can do this or this or this or this. I've got piles of literature. I don't know what to do.' Sometimes patients want you to say to them 'Do you want me to decide for you?' Don't just do it, ask them, and sometimes they will say 'Yes please, that's exactly what I want.' It is a matter of empathy and sensing the feeling of what the individual needs, without assuming that because one patient wants the decision made for them the next one will. Again, the people who need a great deal of help in this situation are the patient's relatives and carers.

It can be very tedious to go through a whole series of explanations, say with a woman with a lump in her breast, and for her husband to turn up at the surgery the next night and want you to go through it all over again with him because he is also frightened. He is one of your patients as well, and his fear and his future are I think just as important.

The other point that patients are concerned about is dignity. This is par-ticularly important in hospital. It is not often that you go into general practices these days where, because the walls are so thin and the place is so crowded, you can actually hear the GP asking the patient behind closed doors 'How's your waterworks?' Such occurrences were once quite commonplace. I hope you all have wonderful premises now and it doesn't happen. However, sometimes we are told that receptionists can be remarkably indiscreet in some crowded settings, where people have sat listening avidly to conversations about other patients which they thoroughly enjoyed, although they were obviously worried that the same thing might happen to them.

The other area that worries people a great deal is lack of concern for the dignity of the elderly. I have to say that standards for the elderly are shamefully low. It is an indictment of the NHS when its very first users are concerned about the standard of their treatment. When your patients, especially those who are elderly, go into care or into hospital, you must be aware of the fact that although they are in someone else's care they still need you. We receive many calls from people whose elderly relatives have become confused when in hospital. A recent example is an 89-year-old who was fine and had had no problems at all before being admitted to hospital for investigation of some rectal bleeding. She then became disoriented, stopped drinking properly and became dehydrated, but no one noticed and made her drink liquids. When her food came she could not reach her tray because it was dumped in front of her and nurses do not feed patients any more. She developed malnutrition and dehydration, and she became totally confused and disoriented. The nurses put up a drip, which frightened her even more. In the end her daughter was in despair. If only her GP had called once to see what had happened to his patient and, knowing what this patient had been like before he admitted her to hospital and seeing what had been done to her, he might have been able to intervene. The older patients particularly need you when you send them to hospital for any reason, because the above type of scenario occurs much too often.

Carers are people as well, and it is terribly easy to slip into the pattern of thinking that really they are part of the network of care, and treating them like a colleague, which is what we want – but they are patients, too.

Finally, we need to feel that the service which patients receive is really tight-knit, with no holes in it for them to fall through. We desperately need the right communication between the doctor and the hospital. Patients need to know that there is a system there for them to contact someone for advice. For example, for a patient who has to attend the day-surgery unit this may seem a great idea until, say, they have had some sort of 'gynae' procedure and subsequently, when they are back at home, they wake up in the middle of the night bleeding, frantic and frightened. They need to speak to someone then and there about what might have happened during the day, when they had their operation, when they were sent home and everything was all right. Perhaps with the advent of NHS Direct the situation is now somewhat better, and the above scenario is certainly an example of an area where NHS Direct might help.

Patient views

The Patients' Association thought that the National Patients' Survey would help to provide information about what people want from the health service. However, when they come up with 12 million forms to be completed in four days – three things that would improve the health service, and only a small space to write in – that is politics!

The Patients' Association wants a real survey, and it is going to try to conduct one when it has the financial resources. All I am giving you here is a snapshot that comes from the helpline. It is thought that primary care groups (PCGs) and primary care trusts (PCTs) will help. The Patients' Association is a little nervous about the fact that there is only one lay member on the Board of each PCG, and we have evidence that by and large this lay member is tending to be a local councillor. You need liaison groups of your own patients, and I know that some GPs have achieved that. The Patients' Association tries to help people to set up liaison groups where they want to (tea and biscuits once a month, and suggestion boxes). If you are prepared to take the occasional insult, they can be very helpful. I would very much like to see more in the way of consensus conferences for patients around the country, for the National Institute for Clinical Excellence (NICE) to take into consideration.

Finally, may I suggest that you take a look at the 'fringe'? Vast sums of money are pouring out of your patients' pockets into the pockets of aromatherapists, reflexologists, iridologists – you name it. What are these patients paying for? They are paying for time, I think, which is the hardest thing of all for you to provide – or it seems to be. They pay someone who will listen to them. There is also a lot of touching. Physical touch has enormous importance, and I sometimes think that the GP who remembers to shake hands with every patient can do far more good than he or she realises. You dare not hug patients any more – those days are gone. However, the complementary therapists are offering something, and I believe that you have so much more to offer.

2

Enhancing the quality of general practice through patient feedback

Michael Greco

Introduction

There is increasing pressure to involve users/patients/consumers in the evaluation of health services. The new NHS Plan[1] highlights the importance of users providing feedback to clinicians, managers and other staff about their experiences of the healthcare system. General practice is no exception. The quality agenda is a jigsaw of new policies, including concepts such as revalidation, clinical governance, quality team development (QTD) and continuing professional development (CPD). Each of these quality initiatives stresses the importance of patient feedback.

In the past, patient feedback has been occasional, sometimes critical and mostly supportive, but never thoroughly or systematically gathered and analysed. Not surprisingly, many busy general practitioners have tended to give it a low priority and a wide berth.

How can patients' views be captured, evaluated and incorporated in the quality agenda?

There are two instruments, the Doctors' Interpersonal Skills Questionnaire (DISQ) and the Improving Practice Questionnaire (IPQ), which are being utilised by general practitioners and their staff across the UK in order to enhance the quality of their services.[2] The experience of several hundred GPs strongly indicates that, with proper processes, patient or user feedback can be embraced constructively and with positive outcomes for service quality and user/carer relationships.[3]

Doctors' Interpersonal Skills Questionnaire (DISQ)

The DISQ is designed to give general practitioners structured patient feedback on their interpersonal skills within the consultation. This instrument was designed according to a number of factors, including a review of the international literature, and input from doctor and patient focus groups.[4,5] It is currently being used in the UK as well as in New Zealand, Ireland and throughout Australia as a tool for quality assurance and professional development.

The practice receptionist administers the DISQ to 50 consecutive patients. It contains only 12 items, which are rated by patients on a 1–5 scale, and it takes about two minutes to complete (*see* Box 2.1). The results obtained from patient responses are aggregated and presented to general practitioners in a graphic format according to various patient characteristics, such as gender and whether the patient saw their usual GP. In addition, comments from patients are provided. General practitioners who have undertaken the DISQ have reported that it is 'minimally disruptive'. As a requirement for Post-

---

Box 2.1:   Items contained within the Doctors' Interpersonal Skills Questionnaire (DISQ)

1   My overall satisfaction with this visit to the doctor is...
2   The warmth of the doctor's greeting to me was...
3   On this visit, I would rate the doctor's ability to really listen to me as...
4   The doctor's explanations of things to me were...
5   The extent to which I felt reassured by this doctor was...
6   My confidence in this doctor's ability is...
7   The opportunity the doctor gave me to express my concerns or fears was...
8   The respect shown to me by this doctor was...
9   The time given to me for this visit was...
10   This doctor's consideration of my personal situation in deciding a treatment or advising me was...
11   The doctor's concern for me as a person in this visit was...
12   The recommendation I would give to my friends about this doctor would be...

graduate Education Allowance (PGEA) points, general practitioners complete a brief report after reflecting on their results.

Improving Practice Questionnaire (IPQ)

The development of the IPQ was based on a similar questionnaire used within general practice accreditation schemes in other countries. The questionnaire is structured around commonly agreed standards for general practice (as determined by the Royal College of General Practitioners). The IPQ was further refined after extensive consultations with patients, clinical governance leads in primary care groups and other primary care staff. It has been found to have sound validation properties.

The IPQ consists of 27 items which focus on issues about the practice (e.g. access and availability), the doctor/nurse/PAM (e.g. interpersonal skills), the staff (e.g. manner of reception staff) and finally health promotion activities (*see* Table 2.1). The instrument also provides space for patients to write their comments about how the practice or its staff could improve their service. An example of some of the IPQ items is shown below in Table 2.1.

Table 2.1:   Some items within the Improving Practice Questionnaire (IPQ)

	Poor	Fair	Good	Very good	Excellent
About the practice					
1 Your level of satisfaction with making an appointment	1	2	3	4	5
2 Opportunity to speak to a doctor on the telephone when necessary	1	2	3	4	5
About the doctor (*whom you just saw*)					
11 On this visit I would rate the doctor's ability to really listen to me as...	1	2	3	4	5
12 The doctor's explanations of things to me were...	1	2	3	4	5
About the staff					
21 The manner in which you are treated by the reception staff	1	2	3	4	5
22 Information provided by the practice about its services (e.g. repeat prescriptions, test results, cost of private certificates)	1	2	3	4	5

Utilisation

The DISQ and IPQ are being used in a number of general practice settings, including vocational training, primary care groups as part of clinical governance, and the Royal College of General Practitioners Quality Team Development programme, and there are proposals to use them for revalidation purposes.

Vocational training

The vocational Training Scheme (VTS) in Exeter has conducted a pilot study in which 12 pairs of general practice registrars and their trainers undertook the DISQ as a teaching and learning exercise. After receiving their results with regard to patient ratings (these were sent confidentially and privately in a written format), the registrars and trainers together attended a half-day release educational session to discuss the experience of patient feedback as an individual learning tool and as a basis for registrar/trainer tutorials.

In total, 892 patients completed the DISQ. Based on the calculation that a score of 100% represents all patients rating every DISQ item as 'excellent', the results showed that the mean rating of interpersonal skills for registrars was 80% (range 76–87%). Similarly, trainers had a mean rating of 80% (range 72–87%). Both registrars and their trainers were above the national mean of 77% (based on 500 general practitioners).

Written patient comments were similar for registrars and trainers. Particular comments about interpersonal strengths included 'very understanding, caring and a good listener', 'very friendly, explaining the course of treatment in detail and allaying any fears I had' and 'always approachable'.

Particular comments about areas for improvement included 'to offer me enough time to get out what I want to say', 'sometimes you feel a bit patronised, you feel like you are wasting time' and 'could look more interested in me so that he shows he cares about my needs'.

The general practice registrars and trainers were asked to comment on the usefulness of the patient feedback exercise in terms of its usefulness in improving awareness of one's interpersonal skills (on a scale consisting of 'poor', 'fair', 'good', 'very good' and 'excellent'). For registrars, 20% rated it as 'fair', 40% as 'good' and 40% as 'very good'. Trainers had similar ratings (20% 'fair', 50% 'good' and 30% 'very good'). These evaluations of the patient feedback experience are similar to the findings of a much larger study on 300 registrars in Australia (*see* Figure 2.1).

Other comments from GP registrars and trainers included the following: 'I now better understand whether patients were satisfied with my consultation style or not. Most of them are happy, but I need to work on letting patients

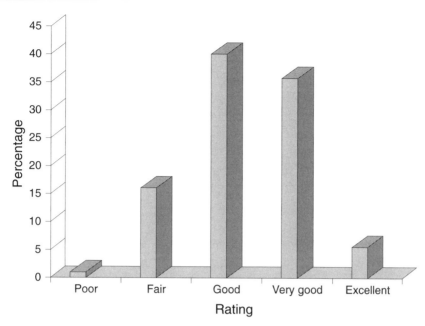

Figure 2.1:   Registrars' ratings of the usefulness of patient feedback in improving awareness of their interpersonal skills.

express their fears/concerns more' and 'The results were encouraging for me personally'. Others commented that 'There was an interesting difference in results between "my own patients" and patients "I do not usually see", as well as a difference between male and female patients' and 'I realise that I remain unable to be all things to all people'.

Trainers were asked to comment on the exercise in terms of its usefulness as part of general practice registrar teaching. Generally, the results showed that trainers found that the feedback provided them with an interesting database on which to raise issues about communication skills. After attending the VTS workshop, several trainers noted that their tutorial sessions would have been more effective if they had had more background information about the exercise. That is, the workshop's content helped them to appreciate more the quality and usefulness of the patient feedback exercise. In some cases, the registrar performed better than the trainer. However, this did not appear to pose any difficulties in the trainer–learner relationship.

In summary, both general practice registrars and trainers valued the experience of patient feedback. It helped them to identify personal strengths and weaknesses, and it provided useful information for registrar–trainer discussions.

Primary care groups

The IPQ has been implemented in over 80 general practices throughout the UK, involving a number of PCGs and covering over 15 000 patients. The results are distributed at three levels – to individual general practitioners, to the practice and to the PCG.

General practitioners have found that the results provide useful insights into their communication skills. Practices have used the results to plan changes in the delivery of their services. In some instances, practice staff are partnering a small group of patients to help them to identify priorities for change based on the overall patient survey. PCGs are also beginning to use the aggregated results of their practices to plan for future training and quality improvement initiatives as part of the clinical governance agenda.

One of the most interesting findings to date is that the patient scores for the interpersonal skills of the general practitioners are much higher than their scores for other aspects of the practice's services (e.g. appointment-making, manner of reception staff, information, etc.). It is obvious from these findings that practices could improve the quality of their services from a patient's perspective by focusing on issues of access, availability and information-giving.

The RCGP's Quality Team Development (QTD) Programme

The IPQ is one of the patient feedback options which practices can choose in order to fulfil the QTD requirement for assessing user views about the practice.

The QTD initiative is a quality scheme aimed at helping PCGs develop clinical governance. A local assessment team (which includes GPs, practice nurses and practice managers) assesses practices against criteria drawn from sources such as the General Medical Council's *Good Medical Practice*, college assessments, patient groups and national service frameworks. The local assessment team provides feedback and helps practices to create a practice development plan. Patient feedback will be a useful database enabling the assessment team to monitor the performance of a practice, and to suggest areas for improvement if necessary.

Revalidation

Recently, the DISQ was part of the RCGP's Accredited Professional Development (APD) pilot study. The RCGP intends to make this package available to all GPs as a way of fulfilling the requirements of revalidation. Most of the GPs in the pilot study found the experience of patient feedback on their inter-personal skills to be a very relevant and interesting exercise. It was noted that such feedback is at the hub of general practice, since its focus is on the quality of the patient–doctor relationship. For all concerned, the experience identified some professional and/or personal areas on which to focus in order to improve their interpersonal skills.

Having reflected on the feedback from patients, general practitioners were asked to comment on those aspects of their interpersonal skills that required some improvement. Particular comments included the following: 'It appears that I need to improve upon warmth of greeting, explanations and reassurance, especially with patients who are not my usual patients, and females' and 'I need to give more time, share management options, confirm understanding, elicit patient beliefs and explain more fully'. Others commented that 'The main areas for improvement are setting people at ease, not hurrying them, and allowing them to express their concerns and fears', 'Dealing with other doctors' patients, male patients, time given, and second half of the consultation. I should also benefit by improving my self-awareness' and 'Time management, house keeping (i.e. getting ready for each patient) and more on showing empathy'.

Next steps

Obtaining feedback from patients through instruments such as the DISQ and IPQ is only the first step in the quality improvement cycle. Such data acts like a mirror. It highlights one's strengths and deficiencies. Although it is merely a first step, it can not be underestimated, as the process of receiving feedback can be perceived as threatening by some general practitioners and their practices. A cultural shift is still needed if patient feedback is to move from 'rhetoric to reality'.

The next step is to set up strategies for acting on these results. The work-shop participants raised the importance of this action phase. For example, if a general practitioner scores poorly on his or her interpersonal skills, what should be done? Should the doctor discuss his or her results with a colleague? If so, who should this person be? A general practitioner tutor? A clinical governance lead? Another trusted general practitioner? A trusted patient? How can the general practitioner incorporate such feedback into their personal development plan? These are questions which need to be addressed if CPD is to have an impact on quality within the profession.[6]

In Australia, over 2500 GPs have undertaken patient feedback on their interpersonal skills. Many of them wanted some form of distance-learning package which could assist them in further refining their interpersonal skills within the medical consultation. As a result, a workbook/video was developed entitled *Doctors Advancing Interpersonal Skills (DAIS)*.[7] The module consists of a 90-minute video and a 40-page workbook, which includes a number of reflective exercises on communication skills and attitudes.

Conclusion

Eliciting patient feedback and user views are at the heart of the new NHS. The DISQ and IPQ are useful instruments for assisting GPs in a variety of settings and requirements, which represent the jigsaw of general practice.

References

1   Secretary of State for Health (2000) *The NHS Plan – a Plan for Investment: a Plan for Reform.* Department of Health, London.

2   Greco M (2000) Patient questionnaire gives PCGs quality feedback about services. *Primary Care Rep.* **2**: 29–30.

3   Greco M and Brownlea A (2000) Patient input accentuates the positive. *Doctor.* **13 July**: 42–3.

4   Greco M, Brownlea A and McGovern J (2000) Consumers as educators: implementation of patient feedback in general practice training. *Health Commun.* **12**: 173–93.

5   Greco M, Cavanagh M, Brownlea A and McGovern J (1999) Validation studies of the Doctors' Interpersonal Skills Questionnaire. *Educ Gen Pract.* **10**: 256–64.

6   Valentine MJ and Howard JC (2000) *Vision 2000: Managed CPD in the New NHS.* National Association of GP Tutors, Aberdeen.

7   Brownlea A, Buckley B, Field D, Francis W, Greco M and McGovern J (1999) *Doctors Advancing Interpersonal Skills (DAIS): a Workbook/Video Educational Program.* Client-Focused Evaluations Program.

Further information

Further details about the DISQ and IPQ can be obtained from the author at Exeter and North Devon NHS Research and Development Support Unit, Noy Scott House, Haldon View Terrace, Exeter EX2 5EQ.

Part 2

Best evidence medical education

General practitioners involved in undergraduate, postgraduate and continuing education will benefit from combining their teaching and professional judgement with the evidence available in order to decide the most appropriate action in a particular situation. Importantly, the adoption of best evidence medical education does not require the teacher to be a researcher in medical education. Best evidence medical education has much to offer the profession.

David Wall challenges us to emulate the evidence-based practice approach and to apply the same rigour to the medical education field. He challenges the view that education is too soft a subject to supply real evidence for what is done, and he explains how qualitative and quantitative research evidence can be graded.

3

Best evidence medical education

David Wall

> The implementation, by teachers in their practice, of methods and approaches to education based on the best evidence available.[1]

What is it all about?

Medical teachers are trained to make medical decisions based on evidence, but when it comes to teaching, many of them abandon all this and base everything on tradition and intuition. This has been described as the PHOG method, based on prejudices, hunches, opinions and guesses.[2] We hope that, in the future, medical teachers and learners and their institutions will be trained to make educational decisions based on real evidence. Can we obtain real evidence for what we do? Is education so soft a field of work that there is no evidence? Some have advocated the double-blind randomised trial as the only way to test out and gather evidence for educational initiatives, as occurs in studies of new drugs and treatments. Others have suggested that this is illogical, and that to demand evidence based on randomised trials for many issues in education is not feasible.[3] We need to include both quantitative and qualitative research, so that nothing is counted out before we start. The point is that we need to ask what is the best way of answering a particular question. Even Sackett himself has now recanted his previous dogmatic support of the randomised controlled trial, and has suggested that attempts to choose a best overall design involve oversimplification.[4]

The aim of best evidence medical education will be to seek out and grade the power of evidence for medical education innovations and interventions, so that we are able to choose and use the best ones for our purposes.

What do we need to do?

Six steps have been identified in the practice of evidence-based teaching:

- framing the question
- developing a search strategy
- producing the raw data
- evaluating the evidence
- implementing change
- evaluating that change.

Therefore we shall need to appraise the literature critically, and to categorise the power of the available evidence. We shall inevitably identify gaps and flaws in the existing literature, and therefore we will need to suggest (and even conduct) studies to help to address these.

What will be the results of best evidence medical education?

Everyone will be a user of evidence. This will mould the policies and practice of teaching and learning in ways that do not exist at the present time. However, most of us will not need to conduct the reviews or carry out the research work ourselves. Nevertheless, an understanding of the principles and practice of best evidence medical education is important.

What are the problems?

There are problems in getting best evidence medical education accepted by authorities and institutions. For example, over 30 years ago a randomised trial demonstrated the superiority of tapes/slides over lectures.[5] Yet this and other research on the use of lectures has done little to dampen the enthusiasm for lectures in medical education!

There are also problems with the funding of this work. Again, directors of research and development appear to prefer the randomised controlled trial design as the only valid research method, so educational researchers struggle to get the message across.

A change in the culture is needed. When medical teachers make clinical decisions, they do so on the basis of the available evidence, but when they are teaching, many of them abandon the principles of critical thinking, and do not even ask what works and what does not.

Best evidence medical education – the beginnings

Many of us are familiar with the Cochrane Collaboration of evidence-based medicine and reviews of evidence, meta-analyses and randomised trials of various medical treatments. In a similar vein, there are the beginnings of a series of reviews in the areas of evidence-based healthcare, evidence-based policy and practice, and in the fields of education, social science and criminology. These systematic reviews of the effects of social and educational interventions are part of the Campbell Collaboration.[6]

We must remember that medical education involves teaching and learning by adults, and as such should be based on the principles of adult education. Here learners learn best by actively constructing knowledge and understanding in and through their daily activities. Remember Brookfield's six principles of adult learning.[7] These six principles are listed as follows:

1   voluntary participation
2   mutual respect
3   collaboration
4   reflection
5   critical reflection
6   nurturing.

It is about problem-solving, the role of experience, and self-directed learning with a mentor or teacher. Learning tasks should take place in a democratic environment.

Best evidence medical education – some examples

One example of this is the work on the evaluation of problem-based education in the medical schools of McMaster in Canada and Newcastle, New South Wales, in Australia. They have some lectures and seminars, but a great deal of small group work, private study and personal tutorials. There is some evidence that this results in higher levels of student satisfaction and better evaluations, as well as better clinical performance.[6]

Another example is a recent review of teaching communication skills.[8] This article reviewed the work in this area and gave a quality grading of articles. The conclusions were as follows.

•   Communication skills can be taught.

- They are learned.
- Skills are best maintained by practice.
- Teaching should be experiential, not instructional.
- Contents should be problem-defining.
- The least good students improve the most.
- Men take longer to learn than do women.

In the future, we hope that further expert reviews on key topics in medical education will be published for all to see. At the moment, however, we are at the very beginning of this process.

In conclusion, we need to seek out the best evidence for medical education.[9] This involves three key tasks:

1 preparation of systematic reviews of suitable rigour and merit
2 dissemination of the results of this work
3 nurturing of a culture of respect and value for medical teaching equal to that for other aspects of professional practice.

How do we evaluate the different evidence?[10]

We need more research on these issues, so we have agreed what we are going to do, what the definitions are, and that we are working to the same standards. Effectiveness must be linked to outcomes. One way to look at this is to use the Kirkpatrick hierarchy. In a modified form, this may be described as shown below, with five levels of effectiveness:

1 healthcare outcomes
2 health professionals' behaviours, performance and practice
3 learning or knowledge
4 participants' views
5 participation or completion.

To amplify this Kirkpatrick hierarchy, a simple example may help us to understand it a little better. As we know, low-dose aspirin helps to prolong life in patients who have angina, and in those who have had a previous heart attack. There is plenty of evidence to support these claims, but it is not possible to go into this in any detail here. Let us suppose that we wish to construct educational events to get these facts across to doctors and nurses, so that we may have an effect on these groups of patients. How does this fit with the Kirkpatrick hierarchy?

Level 5, participation or completion, would look at those who had completed a course of teaching and learning in this area. We could record the numbers of doctors and nurses who had attended the course, and measure something of the coverage of doctors in every practice in the area. Here we are recording who attended, not whether the course was any good, or whether anyone learned anything!

Level 4, participants' views, would be an evaluation of the programme. What did the participants think of the course? What did they like best and what did they like least about it? Here we are asking whether the participants thought that the course was a good one. It is one step up from just measuring who attended, but still we have no idea whether anyone learned anything, or even put it into practice!

Level 3, learning or knowledge, would evaluate whether the course participants actually learned anything. Perhaps we could have tested factual knowledge before and after the course with a multiple-choice test, or used an objective structured clinical examination (OSCE) before and after the course, and compared the results. We may even have been able to show that the candidates' knowledge did increase after the course! So this is one more step up from an evaluation of the course by the learners, but it still does not look at whether the doctors and nurses went away and put their knowledge into practice when dealing with patients!

Level 2, health professionals' behaviours, performance and practice, would look at whether the participants went back into practice and did in fact identify their patients in these at-risk groups, and put them on low-dose aspirin if they were not already taking it, or adjust the dose of those who were taking the wrong dose. To investigate this would require an audit of patients on aspirin before the course, and another say six months later, and a comparison of the results. Hopefully the second study would show more patients than the first. Thus we have taken another step up the hierarchy, and we have been able to demonstrate a change for the better in the performance of these doctors and nurses in this area.

Level 1, healthcare outcomes, is the highest level of the Kirkpatrick hierarchy. It looks at what actually happens to the patients. Here we would hope that over time our best efforts in prescribing low-dose aspirin would have a beneficial effect on the survival of these patients. This is obviously the most difficult element to measure and to demonstrate. It may require a timescale of several years to show an effect, as well as the expert help of our colleagues in public health medicine in collecting and analysing the right data!

From this example it will be clear that not very many educational initiatives do show an effect at level 1 (the highest level). Nevertheless, we should be aiming to look at the effects of our teaching and learning using the highest level we can. At the very least, it means that we should evaluate our teaching and strive to show that new knowledge and skills have been achieved. There is much work to be done here.

Types of studies in medical education

In attempts to look at studies in medical education, and to grade them along the lines of the Kirkpatrick hierarchy, several problems arise. One of these relates to the many different types of educational studies that have been reported in the literature. These include the following:

- experimental studies
- observational studies
- case studies
- ethnographic studies
- experiential studies.

These all need to be defined, with examples. Another problem relates to inter-pretation of the type of category within which a particular study is classified. This is easier said than done, as a recent study we conducted in Birmingham has shown.[11] We were paired off and then asked to categorise various studies from the abstracts of papers that were given to us. We worked independently, and the results were later compared. We produced some level of agreement, but the correlation was not particularly strong.

One tool for the evaluation of evidence, namely the QUESTS criteria (*see* below), has been accepted for evaluating evidence in educational practice.[10] It attempts to look at two main areas of evidence. Three of the criteria look at the power of the evidence available – the quality, extent and strength of the evidence. The remaining three criteria look at the relevance or transferability of the evidence, the utility, the target and the setting. These six criteria are described below.

- **Q**uality. How good is the evidence?
- **U**tility. To what extent can the method be transferred? Can it be adopted without modification?
- **E**xtent. What is the extent of the evidence?
- **S**trength. How strong is the evidence?
- **T**arget. What is the target? What is being measured? How valid is the evidence?
- **S**etting. How close does the context or setting approximate? How relevant is the evidence?

Further work on these six areas is needed to define, explain and agree oper-ational definitions for these criteria if they are to be implemented in practice. Remember that, with six criteria, we recognise that there is no simple truth about best evidence medical education.

Finally, the implementation of best evidence medical education will not be easy. We are at the beginning of a movement to search for the truth about what works best in our own teaching and learning, and to put that into practice. In this way we may be able to improve our teaching, improve the learners' performance, and have an impact on the better healthcare of our patients.

References

1   Hart I (1999) Best evidence medical education. *Med Teacher.* **21**: 453–4.

2   Harden RM and Lilley PM (2000) Best evidence medical education: the simple truth. *Med Teacher.* **22**: 117–19.

3   Norman GR (2000) Reflections on BEME. *Med Teacher.* **22**: 141–4.

4   Sackett DL and Wennberg JE (1997) Choosing the best research design for each question. *BMJ.* **315**: 1636.

5   Harden RM, Lever R, Dunn WR, Lindsay A, Holyroyd C and Wilson GM (1969) An experiment involving tape/slide programmes for lectures. *Lancet.* **1**: 933–5.

6   Davies P (2000) Approaches to evidence-based teaching. *Med Teacher.* **22**: 14–21.

7   Brookfield S (1986) *Understanding and Facilitating Adult Learning.* Open University Press, Buckingham.

8   Aspegren K (1999) BEME Guide No 2. Teaching and learning communication skills in medicine – a review with quality grading of articles. *Med Teacher.* **21**: 563–70.

9   Bligh J and Anderson MB (2000) Medical teachers and evidence. *Med Educ.* **34**: 162–3.

10 Harden RM, Grant J, Buckley G and Hart IR (1999) BEME Guide No 1. Best evidence medical education. *Med Teacher.* **21**: 553–62.

11 Belfield CR, Thomas HR, Bullock AD, Eynon R and Wall DW (2001) Measuring effectiveness for best evidence medical education: a discussion. *Med Teacher.* Accepted for publication.

Part 3

Devolution

This part of the book consists of a comprehensive review of the effects of devolution on postgraduate GP education in Wales, followed by a summary of the discussion that resulted during the UKCRA Workshop. Simon Smail is both the Chairman of UCKRA and also heavily involved as Sub-Dean and Director of Postgraduate GP Education in providing advice to the Welsh Assembly. He not only describes the changes that have occurred, but also poses important questions for the future. Devolution will affect the whole of the UK, and its effects can already be seen in the *UK Guide to the GP Registrar Scheme*. While the policy remains similar, funding is already diverging. Simon Smail's insight into the new *This United Kingdom* raises many concerns.

4

How will devolution affect postgraduate GP education? A year's experience of devolution in Wales

Simon Smail

Introduction

Devolution is now a reality for Wales and Scotland and, with a less certain start, for Northern Ireland as well. Administration of health matters is now in the hands of four separate governments in the UK, and four separate groups of civil servants. In the past there was a considerable degree of 'read-across' between health policy in each of the four countries of the UK, and post-graduate education was broadly similar in each country. But what will the future hold? How will the new powers of the Assemblies affect the arrange-ments for postgraduate education, the funding and indeed the regulation of education?

The experience of one year's devolution in Wales may point to some of the challenges and indeed threats for the future.

The National Assembly for Wales

On 1 July 1999, the National Assembly for Wales assumed its powers from the Welsh Office, following the election in May of the 60 Assembly Members (AMs). A total of 40 AMs were elected to represent constituencies, and a further 20 AMs were elected on a regional basis, with a complicated form of proportional representation determining their election. The result of the election was a surprise to many commentators, representing a 'quiet electoral earthquake'. The Labour party ended up with the largest share of the seats

(28) but with no overall majority, as had been expected. The Labour group formed a government as a minority administration, intending to look for support to Plaid Cymru (the second largest party), the Conservatives and the Liberal Democrats on each issue as appropriate.

The process of choosing the leader of the Labour group (which preceded the election) was highly controversial. Alun Michael, who was strongly supported by the Prime Minister, ultimately won the selection process despite considerable local support for the other main candidate, Rhodri Morgan. After the election, Mr Michael became the First Secretary of the National Assembly.

The Welsh Assembly is responsible for domestic administration in Wales and for the expenditure of the Welsh budget of around £8 billion, received as a block from Westminster. Health service spending in Wales is £2.8 billion.

The Assembly has subject Committees for Agriculture, Economic Development, the Environment, Health and Social Services, Pre- and Post-16 Education and Local Government. In addition, there are four Regional Committees which deal with the interests of the main Regions in Wales. Chairs of these Committees are drawn from across the party spectrum. A number of Standing Committees deal with the technical business of the Assembly. The Legislation Committee is responsible for overseeing the legislative programme of the Assembly, which is now responsible for all domestic secondary legislation in Wales.

It comes as a surprise to many to realise that all National Health Service (NHS) matters in Wales are now dealt with completely separately from those for England. The NHS Management Executive (NHSME) (for England) has no role in Wales, or in Scotland or Northern Ireland. Thus NHSME discussion papers, policy documents, management letters, etc., are not relevant to the Celtic countries, and are not routinely circulated to any NHS staff outside England. Furthermore, with the advent of the Assemblies, most secondary legislation at Westminster (including that for health service matters) no longer applies outside England. The National Assembly for Wales determines its own secondary legislation.

The Cabinet consists of the First Secretary, the Secretaries for each of the main subject areas, and a Business Secretary. It was anticipated that the Cabinet would collaborate with the backbenchers via the subject committees in devising policy. However, in the early days it appeared that the cabinet was adopting a governing role, with backbenchers left to exert their influence as and when they could.[1] In part, this appeared to be the background to a major upheaval in the affairs of the Assembly, when on 9 February 2000 the First Secretary faced and lost a vote of no confidence. Lord Dafydd Elis Thomas, the presiding officer of the Assembly, opined after this vote that '*this is the first day of devolution*'. Feelings had been running high over the way in which the First Secretary had taken control of the agenda of the Assembly up to that point. Rhodri Morgan was then appointed First Secretary, and announced that he was determined to uphold the key issues of democracy, openness and a consensual approach to policy-making.[2]

Prior to the advent of the Assembly, Civil Servants were mainly concerned with administrative duties, but now they are more heavily involved in policy development, supporting the Cabinet and the Subject Committees. It is clear that the burden of responsibilities, not to mention the workload, of the Civil Service in Wales has broadened considerably. There have been concerns that the expanded role has reduced the ability of the Civil Service to continue to deliver the administrative functions which are still extant.

Indeed, there have been quite serious concerns during the first year of the Assembly over its capacity to deal with the workload, particularly that relating to secondary legislation. The number of items of secondary legislation dealt with during its first year was only a fraction of the number dealt with in the previous year in Westminster and signed off by the Secretary of State for Wales. Thus there is some risk of a legislative 'vacuum' appearing.

How have health issues been addressed in the Assembly?

Health matters are largely in the hands of the Health and Social Services Committee. It should be noted that the Committee deals with both Health and Social Services – this is important in terms of service planning and 'joined-up working'. The overall direction for the Committee is described in the major policy document produced by the Assembly in May 2000, *Betterwales*.[3]

This Committee has set out the following policy priorities for 2000:

- joined-up working in the health services
- improving health and tackling inequalities
- primary care ('a realignment of NHS priorities in the form of a strategy for primary care (health and social), including its contribution to social exclusion and community development')
- quality regulation/inspection
- children
- urgent policy and operational issues
- budgeting.

An 'NHS Stocktake' exercise was undertaken in 1999, and the Committee then set out a programme to develop new areas of NHS provision in line with its own priorities. Early examples include a special allocation of resources for children's services, and also a scheme for free eye tests for a broader section of the population than is entitled to them in England.

After the Spring 2000 Budget (UK), the Assembly was allocated an additional grant of some £80 million for health expenditure. The Health and Social Services Committee will be deciding how this is to be spent. On 13 June 2000 the Health and Social Services Secretary announced that £7.9 million of these funds would be spent on work-force development. Over £2 million has specifically been allocated to improve GP vocational training. Additional GP training posts would be funded, as well as schemes to offer enhancements to vocational training provision. This announcement is in advance of any such consideration in England, and it follows a period of lobbying by the Department of Postgraduate Education for General Practice, the Course Organisers for Vocational Training in Wales and the Royal College of General Practitioners (RCGP) Welsh Council, all of whom have separately met the Health Secretary.

Potential advantages of devolution for postgraduate education for general practice

The process of government of the Assembly is now remarkably open. All papers for the Assembly are published on the World-Wide Web, and AMs have continual access to an intranet and email, both at their offices and at their seats during business in the debating chambers. The Assembly debates are all broadcast live on television. This leads to an increase in potential for lobbying by many voluntary and professional organisations (e.g. the British Medical Association, RCGP, etc.) and by the Postgraduate Deanery. We have already seen the fruits of such lobbying.

Priorities for government health spending will be determined locally, and the Health and Social Services will be open to lobbying. It is also of note that two of the AMs are doctors (both general practitioners), and they are both members of the Health and Social Services Committee. One of these doctors has been a member of the Welsh Council of the RCGP over a number of years, and the other has been heavily involved in the work of Local Medical Committees.

A new formal liaison committee has been set up between the Postgraduate Deanery and officers of the Assembly. In addition, members of staff of the Postgraduate School would be afforded direct access to the Health Secretary on important issues.

In Wales, the position of high priority that is enjoyed by primary care should assist in driving the funding of primary care educational initiatives.

Threats

Some threats also exist. Devolution is not yet dynamically stable, and there have been some delays in implementing budgets caused by hung chamber (e.g. Plaid Cymru delayed agreement on the Health Budget to force a debate on free eye tests). The volume of secondary legislation that the Assembly has passed in 2000 is considerably less than that passed for Wales in 1999. The Civil Servants are heavily stretched in dealing with the business of the Assembly.

Most importantly, perhaps, the changes in priorities may lead to major divergence in NHS functions compared to other parts of UK (e.g. Social Services may gain at the expense of the NHS). It is still not clear how much the Welsh NHS will diverge from NHS services in other parts of the UK. At present, NHSME discussion and policy documents are not circulated in Wales, and Welsh Civil Servants are no longer routinely monitoring all aspects of policy in the NHSME. So, for example, the NHSME consultation paper entitled *Supporting Doctors, Protecting Patients* has not been issued in Wales, and does not apply. However, the Assembly is intending to issue a consultation paper on similar topics, and officials have been holding a series of open meetings throughout the Principality canvassing views on quality issues in medicine. It is clear that the Welsh consultation paper will be very different to that issued by the NHSME.

Conclusion

It is perhaps too early to pass any definitive judgements about the opportunities and threats of devolution. Yet it is clear that those involved in postgraduate education in Wales will have to keep a close eye on UK-wide issues, and also maintain a watching brief on the activities of the Assemblies. Active lobbying will no doubt be required, as well as an ability to respond quickly with proposals for initiatives.

Workshop discussion

Following presentation of the paper, Dr Agnes McKnight, Director of Post-graduate General Practice Education, Northern Ireland, described the present state of devolution in Northern Ireland. The power-sharing executive has 120 members, representing all shades of political opinion in the Province. Arrangements for the delivery of healthcare are quite different at present to those in other parts of the UK – fundholding still exists in general practice, and there is little discussion about revalidation. The Health Secretary has not yet published any clear health strategy.

Professor Stuart Murray, Director of Postgraduate General Practice Education, West of Scotland, then briefly described the situation in Scotland. The Scottish Parliament, with 129 members, has more extensive powers than the Welsh Assembly but has a similar committee structure. The early life of the Parliament had been dominated by debates over education, such that health issues had not been considered in the depth that had been expected.

The healthcare system in Scotland is also quite different to that in England. Primary care trusts manage primary care services in a locality, and seven such trusts exist in the West of Scotland. Local healthcare co-operatives (LHCCs) are the equivalent of primary care groups in England (there are 42 LHCCs in West Scotland).

Professor Murray felt that there was a more distant relationship between Deaneries and the Parliament than was the case in Wales. In part this is a result of the presence of the overarching Scottish Council for Postgraduate Medical and Dental Education, which does have a closer relationship with the Parliament.

Further discussion suggested a number of key themes which will be relevant to the development of Postgraduate Medical and Dental Education (PGMDE) in all countries in the UK.

- It will be important for Deaneries to monitor the development of service delivery organisations within the country in which they operate, to look for links with primary care organisations, and to forge alliances for joint working for the development of both VTS and CPD.
- Support of the service is essential for the development of PGMDE, and training and education provision should be relevant to the needs of the service.
- One must recognise that service patterns will diverge in each of the countries of the UK. Individuals who have responsibility for the development of policy for general practice or for delivering education in general practice must respect differences in approach in each of the four countries.
- Professional standards must be protected across the UK.
- Notwithstanding the need to maintain standards, there is a risk that the drive towards a consensus view may diminish legitimate professional debate.

References

1   Osmond J (1999) *Devolution: a Dynamic, Settled Process?* Institute of Welsh Affairs, Cardiff.
2   Osmond J (2000) *Devolution Relaunched.* Institute of Welsh Affairs, Cardiff.
3   National Assembly for Wales (2000) Betterwales.com. National Assembly for Wales, Cardiff (http://www.betterwales.com).

Part 4

Information management

In this part of the book, Trefor Roscoe, the well-known authority on information technology, reflects on information management in primary care over the last five years, describes the major changes that have occurred and identifies some of the missed opportunities. He discusses current problems and finally speculates about the possible future developments in information management.

5

Medical knowledge architecture: a new discipline for the twenty-first century

Trefor Roscoe

History – five years ago

In 1995 medical computing was just beginning to have an impact on primary care. Nearly half of all GP practices had some sort of computer, and paperless practices were beginning to appear.[1] Using a computer in the consultation was possibly thought to help to improve clinician performance, but consultations took longer.[2] Most GPs did not use a computer at all, much less so in the consultation. Secretaries still had manual typewriters, and paper-based notes and letters were the main method of recording clinical information. Card indexes were used for conducting audit, but well-kept card indexes with useful morbidity data were rare, even in academic and teaching practices.

The debate on information management in primary care began,[3] and people then started to look at protocols and disease management tools. Nurses in their chronic disease management role started to contribute to the information culture within the practice. Although the Internet was a growing force in America, very few doctors in the UK outside the universities had heard of it. The first dial-up bulletin board for discussions between general practitioners (Pri-Marie Care) was used by a handful of the technophiles. Few doctors in general practice understood the concept of evidence-based medicine, and those who wanted to access journals or perform a literature search had to go to a postgraduate library. Even if the general practitioner knew how to perform a literature search, the librarians often insisted that they were the only people who could have access to the computers. There was no established culture of information assessment, and asking other colleagues meant a chat at a Postgraduate Education Allowance (PGEA) meeting or else telephoning them for advice; email was unheard of.

Since 1995, most general practitioners have had some sort of computer installed in their surgeries, and desktop computers have become almost universal. Audit has become more common, and has recently been emphasised through clinical governance.[4] There are now well-developed ways of recording, storing and manipulating clinical and administrative data. About one-fifth of practices record the majority of their clinical data on computer and are therefore potentially paperless. The distinction between noteless and paperless practices has recently been drawn, and is perhaps more important.[5] By the end of 2000, two-thirds of general practitioners will have an Internet connection within the practice, the majority being on their desktop. The computers that are now used are fast, have plenty of memory and storage, and can connect to multiple data sources within their local network or on the Internet.

Missed opportunities

Unfortunately, progress has been delayed. There have been many missed opportunities in relation to training key members of primary care teams to understand information management. A universal clinical system to assist data exchange between general practitioners and between primary and secondary care is a recurring theme, but as yet there is no clear way of implementing this. The experience in Scotland of the GPASS system and widespread NHS net connection has not provided the expected benefits. This appears to have been mainly due to lack of training and also a lack of willingness among GPs on the ground to grasp the nettle of technology.

The political aspiration of electronic health records by 2005 will remain just that unless the issue of how to encode and classify clinical data in primary care is addressed. The Read code system could have been a significant and exciting force in clinical information management. Read codes were intended to offer a simple system for clinical data entry. However, the simplicity was lost during the overdiversification of the Read system in an attempt to capture all of the conditions and nuances of healthcare. That system has also suffered from the lack of general support from rank and file, although integration with SNOMed and proper training coupled with a wider understanding of what they could achieve may yet save the day.

Another missed opportunity is the implementation of the NHS net, which has been slow and patchy. Poor management, inadequate initial funding and a lack of training have led to incomplete connectivity when completion was predicted. The latest predictions and targets suggest that two-thirds of practices will be connected by April 2001. Until the majority (i.e. over 80%) of physicians and administrators can communicate directly end to end, the system will be barely usable. A mixed economy of telephone, fax, electronic and paper messaging such as we have at the moment creates more work than it saves. The recent decision to fund fully all aspects of NHS net connectivity within primary care will help, but there are still some genuine and persisting concerns about security that require further thought. Little has changed since my review was published in February 1999.[6] The Regulation of Investigatory Powers Bill which threatens to prevent encryption unless the decryption key is revealed to a supposed 'trusted third party' (such as the Government) may yet make matters much worse.

The information and knowledge revolutions

There has been a knowledge revolution in medicine, and this has four aspects. Firstly, there has been the information explosion which has transformed the amount and quality of information that is available to all physicians. Secondly, there has been a revolution in access to this information, for which the Internet has been mainly responsible. Thirdly, the evidence-based medicine movement has given rise to a wider appreciation of the need for critical assessment of the information behind clinical management. Fourthly, the flow of information has changed direction. Librarians have taken an active role in developing information services and have started to drive information to doctors rather than passively waiting for requests for information and then fulfilling them. This is a recent turn of events, and there will be an increased demand for information experts with proper training in primary care in the near future.[7] The librarians have also helped to drive a shift of emphasis in knowledge access, from being researcher driven to becoming needs or consumer driven. A parallel shift from peer review to systematic review has also occurred as part of this revolution.

The knowledge revolution is continuing, and the new patient-targeted Internet resources are only just starting to drive information to consumers. All of this suggests a shift from the specialist having sole access to and thus control of information, to a more pluralistic distribution of information with empowerment of patients as well as of general practitioners.

The quantity of information is only part of the problem. The quality and understanding of the context of the information are crucial to the correct use of it. Eventually the Internet will come of age and there will be sufficient sifting and sorting of the available information to allow some sense to be made of it all. The new discipline of medical knowledge architecture will be pivotal to this change. An understanding of the difference between information and knowledge, and of how knowledge can be applied and used by expert and non-expert alike will become widespread, leading to a different culture – one that is based on information. It will be the job of knowledge architects to design and build the skeleton on which to hang the body of knowledge, and to implement the access routes to it.

The current situation and the future

It is very puzzling that after 50 years the NHS still does not have a proper information management culture, despite its information requirements. It is not taught to medical and nursing students, and it has hardly penetrated practice management. The local information strategy produced by health authorities will be crucial in determining the direction of information management. It is to be hoped that most local information strategies will pay sufficient attention to the training issues that continue to be a major stumbling block to proper implementation of information management strategies.

One solution to the training issue could be Web-based learning and teaching. The WISDOM project is a beacon for such learning in primary care.[8] By identifying learning goals, collecting links to Web-based information resources and setting up discussion groups to allow peer-to-peer online mentoring, WISDOM has been able to fulfil the learning needs of the participants.[9] It offers a flexible learning experience. Secure and confidential learning environments involving either just two people or the entire group also appear to help the process. Cross-fertilisation between specialities allows new ideas to be created, and the assimilation of these ideas is more rapid than if they had been taught conventionally.

Summary

To summarise this rather eclectic tour of five years of information management in primary care, there has been enormous change and we have come a long way, but we still have a long way to go. We have missed out on some important potential changes that could have been significant to healthcare, such as general practice systems that talked to each other, were integrated with Windows and were easy to use. The Read codes could have been an enormous force in health information management, but instead have stumbled and fallen along the way. We still have massive training requirements, but these could well be fulfilled by the Internet technologies that most people currently regard as the problem rather than the solution. The sheer volume of Internet information overwhelms most people, but once it has been classified and the golden nuggets of information extracted from the morass of useless and misleading data, it will provide the resources that are required for twenty-first century medicine.

References

1 Purves I (1996) The paperless general practice. *BMJ.* **312**: 1112–13.

2 Sullivan F and Mitchell E (1995) Has general practitioner computing made a difference to patient care? *BMJ.* **311**: 848–52.

3 Bryant SL (1997) Practice libraries: managing printed information and meeting the information needs of staff in general practice. *Health Libr Rev.* **14**: 9–21.

4 Scally G and Donaldson J (1998) Clinical governance and the drive for quality improvement in the NHS. *BMJ.* **317**: 61–5.

5 Waring N (2000) To what extent are practices 'paperless' and what are the constraints to them becoming more so? *Br J Gen Pract.* **50**: 46–7.

6 Roscoe TJ and Wells M (1999) NHSnet learning from academia. *BMJ.* **318**: 377–9.

7 Roscoe TJ (1999) Do PCGs need information officers? *Health Libr Rev.* **16**: 129–32.

8 http://www.wisdom.org.uk

9 Fox N, Dolman E, Lane P, O'Rourke A and Roberts C (1999) The Wisdom Project: training primary care professionals in informatics in a collaborative 'virtual classroom'. *Med Educ.* **33**: 365–70.

Part 5

The pre-registration year

The introduction of the pre-registration house officers (PRHOs) to general practice was widely welcomed by general practitioners and educationalists, despite some scepticism from a few hospital consultants in the teaching (but not learning?) hospitals. The initial reaction of GP trainers and the learners themselves has been very positive, but there is a major problem with the scheme – many feel that it is inadequately funded. The initial enthusiasm of trainers has been tempered by the amount of support that the PRHOs require, which is above that of a GP registrar. PRHOs cannot prescribe, and in their first few months they need much help and guidance similar to that required by final-year medical students. Many trainers have warned that despite the educational benefits of the scheme, they are likely to pull out if an enhanced trainer's grant is not forthcoming. We believe that this would be extremely regrettable.

This part of the *GP Jigsaw* provides a unique insight into the development of the scheme from the perspective of a doctor who is responsible for managing the scheme in the West Midlands, and his son, who has recently completed a GP PRHO placement. Alex Heazell, the current PRHO in Stephen Kelly's own practice, has written the Survival Guide, which we thought would be a useful aid to other PRHOs around the country.

6

Pre-registration house officers in general practice: a personal view from the West Midlands

Stephen Kelly

Introduction

In 1944 the Goodenough Committee recommended that the pre-registration year should be the last year of basic medical education.[1] The Medical Act of 1950[2] made the pre-registration year a legal requirement, and the Medical Act of 1978[3] made it possible to undertake part of this year in a general practice setting. In 1987 the General Medical Council produced a booklet encouraging opportunities to acquire experience in general practice during general medical training.[4] The 1997 Primary Care Act eased the requirement that general practice training should be in a health centre, and made it possible to arrange more pre-registration house officer (PRHO) rotations in general practice. The 1997 General Medical Council publication, *The New Doctor*,[5] stressed that:

- the PRHO year is the final year of basic medical education
- this applies to all PRHOs
- all PRHOs need high-quality education and training
- it should be fully implemented by April 2000.

The 1998 Supplement gave details of how PRHOs should learn about patient care in the community setting, and it specified that practices taking PRHOs should be approved training practices with two trainers and having close links with an undergraduate general practice department.[6]

The experiences of organising a general practice PRHO rotation at St Mary's Hospital have been described,[7] and Dr Joe Wilton published a questionnaire study[8] which showed that general practice PRHOs:

- had more teaching in general practice
- spent fewer hours working, but spent more time on clinical activity

- were generally satisfied and would recommend the posts to others
- felt that four months was about the right amount of time to spend in general practice.

He also noted other schemes in Southampton, Liverpool and Cambridge. More recently, a study from North-East England was published on how PRHOs spent half a week in general practice over a four-month period.[9] They reported on how the supervisors required support and possibly further training.

Professor Yvonne Carter and Suzanne Parsons have described how the North Thames region incorporated the St Mary's scheme in 1997 and extended it to 12 four-month posts in rotation with medicine and surgery.[10] They discussed the 1999 input of £41 million from the NHS Modernisation Fund to boost the profile of the profession and address the manpower crisis. They felt that general practice PRHO posts helped to encourage recruitment and would facilitate closer working arrangements between primary and secondary care doctors in the future. They did not consider the financial support to be satisfactory, and they argued that lessons should be learned from under-graduate community-based attachments using Service Increment for Teaching (SIFT).

The West Midland experience

Our experience began in 1997, when all West Midland trusts with PRHOs were invited to submit bids for the pilot. It was stressed that these were new PRHO rotations of four months in medicine, four months in surgery and four months in general practice. We were looking for bids that showed close co-operation between the trusts and training practices that were able to take PRHOs. In addition, we were keen to support areas with recruitment and retention problems. The successful bids were from Birmingham (Heartlands Hospital and City Hospital), Coventry (Walsgrave Hospital) and Dudley (Russell Hall Hospital). Each rotation consists of three four-month slots. All of the slots at Walsgrave were filled with Leicester graduates, one Dudley slot was filled, and three of the six Birmingham slots were filled.

I supervised the pilot in the first year and visited all seven of the first-year post-holders during their general practice component. They were all very happy in the practice, received far more teaching than in hospital, but had some reservations about being separated from their peers and possibly being deskilled in practical procedures. We also had problems with organising con-tracts and finances, the PRHO induction process, the protocol to be used for assessment, and the way in which we organised a support structure. I have followed up this first year and, of the seven post-holders, three have now been appointed to general practice vocational training schemes, one is on a medical rotation, one is on a paediatric rotation, one is on a surgical rotation and one is working for the BBC.

The associate adviser (known as an area director) with overall responsibility for the area now co-ordinates the PRHO rotation in their patch. Tony Robinson looks after the Black Country, Bob Strachan covers Birmingham and Solihull, and Ian McDonald supervises Coventry and Warwickshire. These area directors are the key links for the trusts, as they know about the availability and suitability of the training practices.

This current year (1999/2000) the number of rotations has been increased to three in the Black Country (Dudley, Sandwell and Wolverhampton), four in Birmingham (City, Heartlands Solihull, United Hospital Birmingham and Good Hope Hospital) and two in Coventry. All of the Coventry slots have been filled with Leicester graduates, four of the 12 Birmingham slots are filled, and five of the nine Black Country slots are filled.

Next year (2000/2001) the number of rotations has again increased, and we have filled eight of the nine available Black Country slots, 12 of the 15 Birmingham slots, and six of the six Coventry slots. In 1999, Birmingham Medical School introduced a 'matching plan' for PRHOs. There was initial concern that the general practice posts would not be filled. This does not seem to be the case, despite adverse comments from some teaching hospital consultants who do not now have a monopoly of PRHOs. The trusts that actively recruited have done well, whereas the trusts that did nothing have had problems.

Highlights

These included the following:

- the huge commitment of training practices to the pilot
- the involvement of most clinical tutors
- the support of most medical staffing departments
- the increase in recruitment to the pilot with the matching plan
- the high level of satisfaction of the post-holders with the general practice component
- the support from health authorities.

Recommendations

These were as follows.

- The assessment of the pilot by Professor Janet Grant should be widely circulated.
- Practices must be properly reimbursed.

- A tutor should be appointed to run a release scheme for general practice PRHOs.
- There should be close liaison before appointment and joint interviews.
- A central deanery database should be kept of general practice PRHOs.
- The trainers acting as PRHO supervisors should have special training and support.

Recruitment and retention issues

In the West Midlands we were pleased to see our numbers of general practice registrars (GPRs) increase from 119 in 1996 to the current number of 142. Unfortunately, if the figures are examined more closely, it can be seen that between 1996 and 2000 the number of UK graduates has actually fallen, as has the number of Birmingham graduates (*see* Table 6.1 and Figure 6.1). The increase has been in other EEC graduates and more markedly in non-EEC graduates.

Table 6.1: Distribution of GPRs by place of qualification and year

	1996	1997	1998	1999	2000
Total number of GPRs	119	104	126	120	142
UK	104	88	100	88	91
Birmingham	36	30	37	26	32
Other EEC	10	7	14	13	17
Non-EEC	5	9	12	19	34

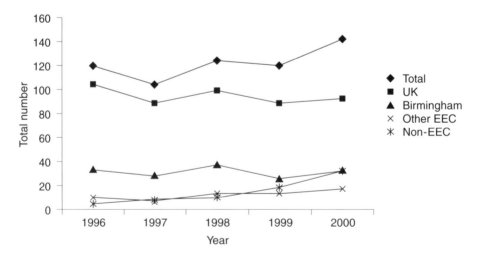

Figure 6.1: Distribution of GPRs by place of qualification and year.

Conclusion

The practices qualifying for the scheme are already extremely busy, in that, apart from the 'day job', they are also committed training practices (with two trainers) and are in some way involved in teaching medical students. We know that this also increases the demands on the practice. To take on a PRHO is a further strain on the practice, thus highlighting the degree of commitment that is needed. This is of course further compounded in deprived areas with higher workloads. I believe that our training practices in these areas are among the best because they can only reach the required criteria by trying much harder. This in turn requires a higher level of motivation. There is a danger that if practices in difficult areas are not supported they will lose heart and give up, resulting in teaching and training being confined to the leafy suburbs (if in general practice at all). This obviously has implications for recruitment to deprived areas.

We need urgent support for this pilot, which was introduced without adequate financial pump priming and which has relied on the good will of general practitioners. The practices that are able to take PRHOs are also under increasing pressure to take more medical students, and at present there is a financial disincentive to take PRHOs. There are excellent educational reasons to encourage PRHOs to spend time in general practice, and in addition there is the prospect of major work-force problems in general practice which could be addressed by supporting the pilot.

The management monies seem to have disappeared into secondary care, and I feel that the input by practice-based administration has been grossly undervalued.

Acknowledgements

I am very grateful to all of the practices and PRHOs that have supported the pilot. The area directors have played a key role, and I am very grateful to them.

References

1   Goodenough W (1994) *Report of the Inter-Departmental Committee on Medical Schools.* HMSO, London.

2   (1950) *Medical Act 1950.* HMSO, London.

3   (1978) *Medical Act 1978.* HMSO, London.

4 General Medical Council (1987) *Recommendations on General Clinical Training.* General Medical Council, London.

5 General Medical Council (1997) *The New Doctor.* General Medical Council, London.

6 General Medical Council (1998) *The New Doctor: Supplement on General Clinical Training in General Practice.* General Medical Council, London.

7 Harris CM, Dudley HAF, Jarman B and Kidner PH (1985) Pre-registration rotation including general practice at St Mary's Hospital Medical School. *BMJ.* **290**: 1811–13.

8 Wilton J (1995) Pre-registration house officers in general. *BMJ.* **310**: 369.

9 Illing J, Taylor G and van Zwanenberg T (1999) A qualitative study of pre-registration house officers in general practice. *Med Educ.* **33**: 894–900.

10 Carter Y and Parsons S (2000) Pre-registration house officers in general practice: opportunities and pitfalls. *Med Educ.* **34**: 248–9.

7

General practice as part of the pre-registration year: the views of a pre-registration house officer involved in the first year of the pilot scheme

Andrew Kelly

As a final-year medical student, along with exams I had the challenge of selecting a PRHO job. At the time I was attached to a vascular surgery firm in Coventry, and I enquired about working for them in the following year. I was told that the job had become incorporated into a rotational scheme with four months of general and vascular surgery, four months of general medicine and four months of general practice experience. I was keen to work for the vascular surgeons and agreed to accept the rotation. At the time of acceptance I was relatively unaware of the role played by a PRHO in general practice

I learned that my job was to be part of a pilot scheme in accordance with the GMC *New Doctor* document. My first four months after qualification were spent at the Walsgrave Hospital in Coventry working, as planned, for the general and vascular surgeons.

In December 1998 I was warmly welcomed to the Allesley village practice on the outskirts of Coventry, where I was to spend the following four months.

A typical day would start at 8.30a.m. with morning surgery, seeing patients on a 'first come, first seen' basis. Once the patients who had come to the practice had been seen, house calls were shared out between the doctors who were working on that day. After lunch and time for private study, I would return for evening surgery, taking house calls either at the beginning or at the end of surgery.

At first I was extremely closely supervised when conducting surgeries. Plenty of time would be allowed for patients, which meant that I could see them without feeling pressurised and I also had time for discussing patients or cases with the supervising doctor. This support was present throughout my stay, although as I progressed the leash was loosened a little to allow me to take more clinical responsibility.

I thoroughly enjoyed my time at Allesley and felt that my skills as a clinician developed in many different ways. While working as a hospital-based PRHO I was able to acquire technical skills relating to the management of patients, all of which are essential to functioning as a junior in hospital. In general practice I was able to concentrate on history-taking, eliciting clinical signs and communication skills – again, skills that are vital to any clinician. I was also able to expand my knowledge of the management of chronic disease. As a junior in hospital, treatment of a patient is often a 'one-off' experience, especially in surgical specialities. A patient will be unwell, undergo a procedure and hopefully be discharged again in good health. In general practice, patients may be seen many times and minor adjustments made to treatment. An obvious example would be the general practitioner's management of hypertension.

I believe that my time in general practice benefited my skills as a clinician, especially as I am currently on a basic surgical training rotation. I may never have the opportunity to work outside hospital medicine again, so a period such as this has been extremely useful.

UKCRA Conference 2000

Workshop on Pre-Registration House Officers in General Practice: conclusions of the delegates

- The patient's perspective should be considered when assessing the pilot.
- On-the-ground feedback from the PRHOs has been good.
- Prescription issues could be addressed by the creation of a limited list of drugs that the PRHO could prescribe.
- Very little of the £41 million from the NHS Modernisation Fund has reached primary care.
- Proper funding for the pilot needs to be guaranteed.
- Funding should reflect that agreed for the placement of final-year medical students in general practice.
- The practices taking PRHOs are already under considerable pressure with clinical commitments, medical student placement and GP registrars. These practices need increased support if they are to continue to survive.

- The promised evaluation from Professor Grant should be made widely available and a decision made on the viability of the pilot study.

Delegates attending the workshop included Dr C Hand, Dr J Hussey, Dr S Kelly, Dr I MacDonald, Dr P Nolan, Dr T Robinson, Dr M Rowan-Robinson and Dr C van Vliet (PRHO in the Dudley scheme).

8

The GP pre-registration house officer survival guide

Alexander Heazell

The job itself

The pre-registration house officer (PRHO) post in general practice is different to most of the experience gained as a student or as a PRHO in other areas. Patients consult with you as their GP, and expect you to function as a knowledge base, prescriber, investigator, gateway to secondary care services and listener.

This is quite a shock to the system, although it becomes much easier after the first few days. Patients will have expectations of you now that you are not only a doctor, but *their* doctor. With the help of your supervisor, your degree and a gradual increase in self-confidence you will be able to deal with 95% of all that is thrown at you with no problems at all.

Differences between primary care and hospital

The PRHO post in primary care differs in many ways from hospital placements, although the magnitude of this difference will depend upon your placement. In general you consult with the patients on your own, and formulate a diagnosis and a management plan which will be reviewed by your supervising GP. Initially the appointments are at 30-minute intervals, which are gradually reduced as you become more proficient. The reviewing procedure promotes discussion and learning about common symptoms encountered within primary care. Currently (2000/2001) the PRHO cannot prescribe without the signature of their supervisor, but in the future it is likely that PRHOs will have a limited formulary.

The first day(s)

The key word for the first few days is *familiarise*. When you arrive at your practice, you will have a GP appointed as your supervisor, who will look after you and your educational needs. It is important to familiarise yourself with the following:

- the practice environment – where are the consulting-rooms, the nurses' rooms, the emergency drugs, etc.?
- the computer system – which buttons do what, what do you need to record and how?
- the medical and nursing staff – you will often see patients who have consulted other GPs, practice nurses or specialist nurses, and their input is invaluable
- the reception and administrative staff – these people will book your surgeries, retrieve notes, file blood results and type referral letters, and you cannot manage without them
- the community healthcare team, including district and Macmillan nurses and health visitors.

Your practice may arrange for you to spend time with other members of the primary healthcare team and administrative staff during your PRHO experience.

Consulting, investigating and referring patients as a PRHO

A wide variety of conditions are seen in general practice. In a four-month period I encountered over 150 separate conditions, ranging from dermatology to orthopaedics. You will learn to consult over a period of time, during which you may deal with other symptoms, conditions and medical problems that affect the patient. Similarly, investigation tends to be more selective and goal-directed than in hospital care. For example, not everyone with a lower respiratory tract infection (LRTI) requires a chest X-ray, FBC, U+E, ESR, CRP, TFTs, glucose, differential WCC, serum rhubarbs, etc.! The consultation may be split over time. For example, a patient with a LRTI may initially require antibiotics, and if there is no improvement or symptoms develop, a chest X-ray may be taken. If this reveals a lesion or you are still unsure, then referral may be appropriate.

Emergencies in general practice

Emergencies in the PRHO post are fortunately few. The following are the most common problems you will have to address in primary care:

- chest pain/angina/myocardial infarction
- acute asthma
- anaphylaxis
- meningitis.

The key message is DON'T PANIC – you will always be supervised. Make sure that you know where the practice keeps the nebuliser and nebules, adrenaline (know the dose) and the emergency bag. If an emergency occurs, get help and call an ambulance (emergency surgery is difficult in a doctor's surgery!). Follow practice protocols (e.g. for anginal chest pain give GTN and aspirin), and wait with the patient.

Important pieces of paper

Patients often attend surgery in order to obtain pieces of paper. These may include exemptions from work, and statutory sick-pay forms (Med 3, Med 4 and Med 5, SC2, all of which have slightly different functions). It is worth reading the attached notes that come with the forms.

Prescriptions may be printed or handwritten, although they are increasingly being computer generated. There are important rules about wording, dose and type of medication, especially with controlled drugs (including opiate-based agents such as methadone). The dose must be written in words (e.g. 75 (seventy-five) milligrams), as must the total quantity (e.g. 28 (twenty-eight) tablets). 'CD' in the *British National Formulary* (*BNF*) indicates controlled drugs.

Requests for death certificates and cremation forms are less frequent than in PRHO posts based in hospital, but they do occur. Once again it is worth reading the notes attached to the forms, and going through your first form with your GP supervisor. It is important that you get this right, as the patient's relatives may also be part of your practice population, they will be distressed at this time and they are also in need of your care.

Education and learning as a GP PRHO

Being a PRHO in general practice is completely different to being in hospital. You will need to be more self-sufficient, and your learning will become more self-directed. The education programme is quite intensive. You will spend a lot of time both with your educational supervisor and with other clinicians (including nurses). This is a golden opportunity to learn about effective consultation skills and to reflect on your own style.

As a PRHO you have to fill in the necessary documentation from your Postgraduate Dean to ensure that you gain full registration from the General Medical Council at the end of your PRHO year. Your supervisor and yourself should meet at 0, 2 and 4 months to assess your progress.

Within general practice, you will have specific tutorials on common diseases, certification, prescribing, etc. You may also be able to sit in on the GP registrar tutorials. In addition, there will be primary care postgraduate meetings which cover a wide range of relevant topics.

There will be a wide range of educational opportunities during your placement. Useful visits include the local hospice, health visitors, funeral directors and crematorium (as relatives will ask questions and expect you to know the answers) and prison medical units.

During the PRHO placement you will be expected to do an audit. It should be small, simple and achievable in four months. This will give you useful audit experience and feedback, as audit is a central part of GP registrar training.

Holidays

There are two important points to bear in mind about annual leave. First, find out whether your annual leave is transferable between your GP and hospital-based blocks, and secondly make sure that you take it – as you cannot look after others if you do not look after yourself.

Finally...

The most important point of all is to enjoy your placement!

Sources of information

www.primarycareonline.co.uk: a great source of information about general practice.

www.bmj.com: BMJ online and a free Medline service to BMA members.

www.rcgp.org.uk: information about general practice training, etc.

www.dss.gov.uk: information for medical advisers with regard to Med 3, Med 4 and Med 5 forms.

Part 6

Vocational training for general practice

The success of the government's *NHS Plan*[1] will depend on a well-trained work-force, and especially on general practitioners, who will have the pivotal role both in providing care for patients and in the management of the new system. However, there is considerable evidence that the recruitment rate is falling[2] and that the education and training of general practitioners have been caught in a time warp.[3] There has been a clamour for changes in the general practice training system to prepare future general practitioners for life in the ever-changing NHS.[4–6]

However, there is also cause for optimism. The way in which general practice training is organised across the UK has changed. In March 2000, Lord Hunt, Minister for Health, launched the new UK GP Registrar Scheme,[7] which should lead to exciting and innovative training opportunities for doctors who want to become GPs. These will include the opportunity to spend a larger part of the training in the primary care setting pursuing a particular learning need (e.g. learning more about the management of drug addiction). The new arrangements will enable the directors of postgraduate general practice education to provide more opportunities for refresher training both for doctors returning to general practice and for those who have trained abroad.

The new UK GP registrar scheme is not the end point. The *NHS Plan* heralded a major review of the senior house officer grade which should deliver a radical overhaul of the hospital component of GP training and lead us into a new era of programme-based learning.

In this part of the book, leading educationalists examine the structure and process of GP vocational training and offer some pointers for a brighter future.

References

1   Department of Health (2000) *The NHS Plan*. Department of Health, London.

2   Medical Practices Committee (1997) *Survey of General Practice Recruitment in England and Wales*. Medical Practices Committee, London.

3   Bain J (1996) Vocational training: the end or the beginning? *Br J Gen Pract.* **46**: 328–33.

4   Hayden J, Styles WMcN, Grant J and Mountford B (1996) Developing vocational training for general practice: a system for the future. *Educ Gen Pract.* **7**(1): 1–7.

5   Elwyn GJ, Smail SA and Edwards AGK (1998) Is general practice in need of a career structure? *BMJ.* **7**: 731–3.

6   Department of Health (1995) *Hospital Doctors: Training for the Future. The Report of the Working Group on Specialist Registrar Training* (supplementary report by the working groups commissioned to consider the implications for general medical practice, overseas doctors and academic and research medicine arising from the principal report). Department of Health, London.

7   Department of Health (2000) *The GP Registrar Scheme. Vocational Training for General Medical Practice: the UK Guide*. Department of Health, London.

9

The regulatory framework for vocational training for general practice in the UK

Justin Allen

Introduction

In this chapter, Europe's leading expert on the regulatory framework of vocational training for general practice explores the issues concerning the current regulatory framework in the UK. He explains the need for a regulatory framework, and then discusses the need for and potential benefits of an overhaul of the current system.

The current vocational training regulations have served the discipline of general practice well, but have for some time been out of date, out of touch with changes in the delivery of healthcare, and restrictive to the further development of good general practice training. There have been increasingly strident calls for their abolition from many groups involved in postgraduate general practice education. However, little thought has been given to what, if anything, should replace them.

The current regulations

The regulations governing vocational training for general practice were first introduced in 1979. They were founded in the medico-political context of the time, and have remained substantially unchanged since then, although some changes were made, first in 1994 to bring UK law into line with the requirements of the European Union Directive on medical training, and then again in 1998 with the introduction of summative assessment.

The Joint Committee on Postgraduate Training for General Practice (JCPTGP) tried to make amendments to the regulatory framework almost as soon as it was implemented, but was unsuccessful.

The case for regulation

There is no doubt that some form of regulatory framework will be needed, if only because European Union (EU) legislation prescribes minimum periods of training to which domestic legislation must conform. EU legislation currently requires a minimum of two years' training in total, only six months of which need be undertaken in a general practice setting. Realpolitik also dictates that some form of managed system will need to be in place if the Government is to agree to provide the necessary funding for general practice training. The Government will legitimately also wish to set limits on professional autonomy and ground rules for professional accountability. The challenge is therefore to produce a framework which satisfies both the desire of the discipline to facilitate development, and that of society and the Government, who will look for cost-effectiveness and the securing of patient safety and service delivery.

What is wrong with the current regulations?

The 1979 regulations still form the basis for the current framework, in that large parts of them have been incorporated into the 1997 version, and they reflect the medical culture of the 1960s and 1970s. However, they were a compromise between the desirable and the achievable. This was the era of the general practitioner being regarded as the failed specialist!

The regulations stipulate the time to be spent, not the skills to be acquired, in a training practice (one year), and the time in hospital senior house officer (SHO) posts approved from a list of specialities and approved by the specialist Royal College (one year). A further year can be spent in any approved training post (this has invariably been a further year of SHO training).

The concept of equivalent experience, introduced in the 1979 regulations, was to allow training undertaken for a career in specialist medicine to count towards the training requirements of general practice. It also allowed more unusual types of experience (e.g. overseas work) to be counted. Its application has been enormously problematic, although it has given the JCPTGP flexibility to exercise its powers, and has enabled it to approve training in innovative posts. However, this flexibility has been greatly diminished by the implementation in 1998 of the Department of Health's Health Service Circular, *The Recruitment of Doctors and Dentists in Training*. This important directive prevents post-graduate medical deans from funding training posts that are not approved by the specialist training authority (STA) and the specialist colleges, even if they are suitable for general practice training. Equivalent experience has therefore become a dangerous loophole which allows doctors with possibly substandard training to be exempted from the summative assessment process – it has out-lived its usefulness.

The training programme is time-based, not competency-based, with a strict envelope of three years' prescribed experience, regardless of the educational needs of the doctor concerned. It is predicated primarily on the service needs of secondary care, and not on the educational requirements of general practice. Thus it has never been truly learner-centred. Training for general practice involves a series of 'posts', with no overall programme of experience required or expected from those 'posts'. The only link between the individual posts is the half-day release course, which is a 'bolt-on' accessory. Two-thirds of the training is therefore not grounded in a primary care setting, and control of that educational experience is to a very great extent outwith the control of the discipline of general practice and its educators. It is remarkable that a system that is so inflexible in meeting the learning needs of individuals with different levels of ability has been so successful. Working within the present regulatory framework, the discipline of general practice has developed a very high-quality training programme.

Amendments to the regulations have been a mixed blessing. The 1994 regulations confirmed the establishment of a generalist competent authority, the Joint Committee, but gave an acquired right in perpetuity for doctors who had no GP training to work as locums or assistants (or in any capacity as a GP in the rest of the European Union).

The 1997 regulations brought in summative assessment as a requirement for all those undertaking a year as a GP registrar, and gave the JCPTGP as the Competent Authority responsibility for supervising all posts used for GP training. However, a major flaw was that it retained the need for the specialist competent authority, namely the specialist training authority, to first approve for specialist training all SHO posts that the general practice establishment would like to use for general practice training.

What do we need from our regulatory framework?

The aim of any new drafting of the Vocational Training Regulations should be to synthesise the conflicting needs of all interested parties. For the patients we must ensure that doctors are trained to be competent primary care physicians who are capable of adapting to the changing needs of the NHS. For the learners we must provide an appropriate educational experience tailored to assess individual learning needs, and not artificially constrained by time or service commitments.

For the general practice educators the regulatory framework should be sufficiently flexible to enable them to provide education programmes tailored to the needs of the doctors in training. Finally, for the health service in all four countries of the UK we need to demonstrate the cost-effective use of valuable resources within a properly accountable framework. This accountability must include quality assurance of the end product.

The regulatory framework must meet the requirements of external bodies such as the European Union, and for the patients' sake we must try to ensure that European regulation is similarly amended. Any new regulatory framework should be flexible enough to develop with the evolving shape of service delivery in primary care, and not take more than 20 years to change!

A future model for medical education for general practice

A future model for medical education for general practice might be as follows. After basic medical education, an extended period of pre-registration house officer work would follow, to include six months of general practice experience for all doctors. Those wishing to enter general practice training would, on appointment, undergo an assessment of their previous experience and learning needs. A teaching programme would be devised which would be tailor-made for the individual. This would include a period of skills acquisition in a secondary care setting, as well as a minimum period of 12 months in general practice.

The total learning programme should be a minimum of two years and not normally more than five years. Flexibility and learner need should be the key determinants. Progression would be determined by at least an annual assessment of progress and, if necessary, by a revision of the education programme and timetable.

Training undertaken for a career in another discipline should not normally exempt a doctor from undertaking all of the general practice training programme. Training to be a cardiologist is not training to be a general practitioner. Specific skills that are acquired during any such previous medical training, whether in the UK, the European Union or overseas, should be assessed and acknowledged when developing a learning plan for an individual doctor.

What should be changed in the regulatory framework?

It is important that some of the key features of the current regulations are retained. I would propose to keep the minimum period of training in general practice at least as long as that specified in Directive 93/16, and probably longer (at least one year). The summative assessment of competence is essential for the protection of patients. A UK generalist competent authority should supervise training and issue certificates to those who are appropriately qualified. If there is to be a general practitioners' register, then the generalist authority should control access to it. An effective appeal mechanism, such as now exists, is also an essential component of any regulatory system.

The naming of the STA or speciality colleges in general practice regulations must be discontinued. From the use of experience (i.e. time in post) as the outcome measure, we must move to purely competence-based outcome measures. Equivalent experience is an anachronism, and should be replaced by an assessment of skills gained.

A new regulatory framework should include increased flexibility in the overall length of training, to a maximum of five years. When appointed, each trainee should participate in the construction of a learning plan setting out objectives and the length of all components of the training programme. The educational placements – either in hospital or in general practice, or indeed in a healthcare setting – should be determined by learning needs and not by service needs. The new regulations should also state explicitly that there should be assessments of educational progression and the opportunity to undergo further periods of training within the overall maximum period specified.

How might this be achieved?

There are a number of changes already in train, and we are experiencing a climate of change in the NHS. The Medical and Dental Education Levy (MADEL) transfer has given the deaneries more flexibility in the delivery of general practice training, and many innovative vocational training schemes are being developed. Plans are already well advanced to develop more stringent appointment procedures, and the creation of an individual learning plan for every appointee is only a short step away.

As announced in the Government's National Plan, the SHO grade is to be reviewed. Doctors who are 'marking time', having completed the necessary number of posts to qualify them for entry to the specialist registrar grade, occupy many posts at this level. However, it is a waste of educational resources for training posts to be occupied in this way. At the same time, service delivery to patients must be guaranteed.

It is important to develop an appropriate strategy to address the legitimate concerns of all parties. The major stumbling blocks will be administrative (finding time to enact the necessary parliamentary regulations) and medico-political (dealing with specialist colleges and the STA).

It is of paramount importance for the whole discipline of general practice – the RCGP, the General Practitioners' Committee, the directors of postgraduate general practice education, the associate directors and the JCPTGP – to work together if anything meaningful is to be achieved. The door is slightly open, so let us place our foot in it and push together!

10

The future of GP vocational training

Simon Smail

Introduction

There is now wide agreement that vocational training for general practice in the UK is outdated and in serious need of a major overhaul.[1] Yet an agreed strategy to carry out a major reform has not yet emerged. Differences of opinion among a variety of lobby groups appear to be holding back attempts to revolutionise the training programme. However, there is now some general agreement on 'next steps' towards a new approach, and there are grounds for optimism that incremental progress will occur. Nevertheless, it will be important to agree a vision for the direction of travel.

The current training programme

The current training programme for general practice – essentially two years in hospital practice and one year in general practice – has remained largely unchanged for two decades. The signs are that it is creaking and failing to deliver an educational experience that provides a cadre of young general practitioners who are 'fit for purpose' in the NHS of the twenty-first century.

What is the evidence that the programme is failing to deliver?

Poor recruitment

If there is evidence of failure in the 'marketing' of an educational programme, questions should be asked as to whether or not the programme is appropriate to the needs of those who might choose to undertake it. (However, there may be many other reasons why young doctors decide not to train for general practice.)

At present there are still difficulties in interesting undergraduate students in a career in general practice. In a study in one medical school, only 14% of male students and 27% of female students planned to enter general practice.[2] However, in order to staff the expected number of vacancies in general practice, around 40% or more of the medical students graduating in the UK should be training for general practice. Lack of recruitment to the vocational training schemes could be viewed as a failure of marketing, and might possibly imply that the training programme itself is inappropriate or else insufficiently relevant.

In Wales we have undertaken a detailed survey of the reasons why current registrars decided to enter the scheme.[3] It appears that when considering which VTS scheme to select, they were most concerned to choose a scheme that offered high-quality teaching in hospital posts. For them, high-quality training in hospital was a major factor determining their choice of scheme. The registrars appeared to take it for granted that they would be offered high-quality training in general practice. Yet their experience showed that the actual experience in SHO posts was not as satisfactory overall as they would have liked. Such findings do illuminate some of the difficulties that are currently being experienced in recruiting doctors to general practice.

Risk of drop-out

The number of young doctors who regret choosing medicine as a career is worryingly high. In a survey conducted in 1996,[4] 68% of SHOs and no less than 80% of GP registrars reported regretting their choice of career at some stage in their training. One must be concerned that the training programme is failing to support doctors who have started down the road of preparation for a career in general practice.

Delay in proceeding to work as a GP

In 1998, only 31% of Welsh GP registrars intended to enter a career post in general practice on completing vocational training, and the majority expected not to enter practice for up to three years.[3] In total, 16% were undecided about whether to enter general practice at all. A survey of the educational needs of new GPs undertaken by Grant[5] in 1998 provides evidence that new GPs do not feel adequately prepared for general practice by their training programme. This would appear, at least in part, to explain the delay in entering practice. Yet further educational opportunities for these doctors who would like to extend their training are meagre. Many of them undertake further SHO posts, which may be of some value educationally and equip them with more clinical skills, but others work as non-principals with variable levels of educational support – which in some cases may be non-existent.

International comparisons

In many countries which have well-developed GP training programmes, the time spent training in general practice exceeds the time spent in hospital practice. Many commentators still find it strange that the balance of time spent in training is so heavily oriented towards hospital-based experience. However, it should also be acknowledged that the type of training that is available in hospital is often not as relevant to the clinical demands of general practice as should be the case. For example, around 10% of consultations in general practice are for dermatological conditions, yet few VTS schemes offer specific training in dermatology skills.

Solutions?

Early experiences

It is pointless simply to plan for changes to the VTS scheme in isolation from other parts of the educational curriculum. Appropriate exposure to general practice in undergraduate training has been shown to influence career choice.[6]

It should be possible to construct an undergraduate curriculum which acts as the beginning of a programme of lifelong learning for general practice.[7] Incorporating appropriate learning models in the early stages could help to lay a foundation for continuing learning in general practice – for example, building on a model such as that described by Slotnick[8] in 1999 (see Figure 10.1).

Early experiences in the PRHO year are also important. Positive experiences at this time and integration with a curriculum that emphasises the principles inherent in general practice patterns of care will have a very beneficial impact.

New approaches to VTS

A number of commentators have suggested a variety of incremental steps to improve the provision of VTS. For example, the GPC Registrars' Subcommittee is particularly concerned to improve the type of hospital post available, and

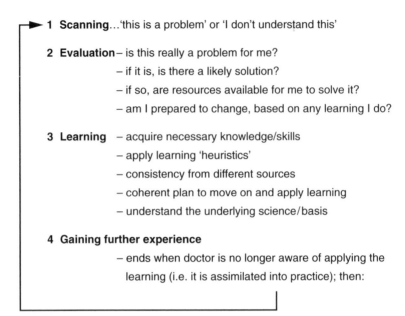

Figure 10.1:   A model for lifelong learning in clinical practice (based on Slotnick).[8]

also to reduce the time spent in SHO posts, so that at least 18 months can be spent in practice. Yet this committee is still pursuing a policy of insisting that it should be possible to train for general practice within a total of three years. This policy is certainly at odds with the groundswell of opinion (including that of the majority of registrars) that a VTS scheme of just three years forms an inadequate basis to provide the full range of knowledge and skills that are expected of a GP principal.

The Royal College of General Practitioners (RCGP) is concerned that vocational training should provide a more flexible approach, based on achievement of skills, knowledge and attitudes, rather than on time served. It argues for regular formative assessment throughout training, and for the availability of a variety of posts at relatively short notice for GP trainees to access as educational needs are identified.

However, the RCGP does acknowledge that there should be a minimum time served. Others are currently arguing for a major overhaul of the SHO grade, with first-year SHOs perhaps undertaking a period of general professional training in two 6-month or three 4-month posts.

The Directors of Postgraduate Education for General Practice in the UK are proposing that the pattern of training for general practice in the future could build on a foundation consisting of a basic set of minimum requirements. It is envisaged that all SHOs would commence their training with one year of general professional training. Ideally this should be in three 4-month posts, but it could be in two 6-month posts. After this initial SHO year, GP trainees would follow a specially identified educational pathway for general practice training, while those intending to pursue a specialist career would enter basic specialist training.

Specific training for general practice would commence after one year in general professional training, and would continue for a further year of SHO-grade posts. However, the training posts in this year would be specially identified or constructed to provide clinical training of specific relevance to general practice. Such posts could be in hospitals or in the community, and would be likely to include experience in out-patient care as a major part of the clinical experience. The posts would also be able to provide hospital-based training in skills relevant to general practice (e.g. in ENT, dermatology, ophthalmology, rheumatology, etc.).

A period of 18 months in general practice as a GP registrar would follow. At the end of training, the GP registrar would complete the MRCGP examination (or summative assessment) and then enter a period of higher professional training. This could be undertaken as a principal or non-principal by day-release over the first two or three years of practice. During this time, an academic programme would be followed, such as a Diploma or Masters course. Some doctors may wish to undertake academic training in a full-time post for one or two years following vocational training. Such posts would be appropriate for those interested in an academic career in general practice, or in developing leadership skills to enable them to take on roles in the management of general practice or advanced clinical practice.

The future?

One advantage of the model proposed by the Directors of Postgraduate Education for General Practice is that it could be implemented incrementally. The Health Secretary in Wales announced the allocation of additional funds to extend and develop vocational training in Wales in 2001. In Scotland, some posts for full-time higher professional education are already available. English directors have made bids to the NHSME for funds to extend the GP component of training on a voluntary basis to 18 months, and have also bid for funds for higher professional education.

There are still many obstacles to overcome in regenerating vocational training for general practice. A clear, consensual vision of the ultimate goal is still needed, and remains somewhat elusive. Patients, educationalists, professional bodies and those involved in making investment decisions for the NHS must all be involved in building a new consensus for the way forward.

A particular difficulty will be faced in modifying SHO posts so that these posts can provide training in those skills that can best be learned in a specialist environment and that will be useful in general practice. A completely new type of SHO post is likely to be required. Advancements on this agenda will only be possible if there is a clear consensus on the importance of providing relevant educational training for GPs, and an acknowledgement that GP SHOs cannot be regarded as providing a large measure of service activity during their placements.

References

1   Elwyn GJ, Smail SA and Edwards AGK (1998) Is general practice in need of a career structure? *BMJ.* **317**: 730 –33.

2   Field D and Lennox A (1996) Gender in medicine: the views of first and fifth year medical students. *Med Educ.* **30**: 246–52.

3   Smail SA (1998) *Current State and Future Aspirations for Vocational Training in Wales.* Department of Postgraduate Studies, University of Wales College of Medicine, Cardiff.

4   Allen I and Jackson N (1996) *The Career Choices of Medical Students and Junior Doctors.* Unpublished paper. Policy Studies Institute, London.

5   Grant J (1998) *An Evaluation of Educational Needs and Provision for Doctors Within 3 Years of Completing Vocational Training.* Joint Centre for Education in Medicine, London.

6   Morrison JM and Murray S (1996) Career preference of medical students: influence of a new four-week attachment in general practice. *Br J Gen Pract.* **46**: 721–5.

7   Hilton S and Smail SA (2001) A lifelong curriculum for general practice? *Educ Gen Pract.* **12**(1): 1–10.

8   Slotnick HB (1999) How doctors learn: physicians' self-directed learning episodes. *Acad Med.* **74**: 1106–17.

11

Enhanced management arrangements

Pat Lane and Fiona Patterson

From 1 April 2000 all costs related to training in general practice in England were transferred out of the General Medical Services (GMS) budget into the Medical and Dental Education Levy (MADEL), and are managed in the deaneries by the Directors of Postgraduate General Practice Education (DsPGPE).

This change is intended to:

1   connect the recruitment, appointment and work-force planning of all training grades in the NHS into a unified management stream
2   increase flexibility within training programmes for general practice
3   ensure the most appropriate training for each individual.

Information previously available within the *Statement of Fees and Allowances (Red Book)* has been revised and published as *The GP Registrar Scheme – Vocational Training for General Medical Practice (The UK Green Guide).*[1]

The NHS is now clearly expected to demonstrate the characteristics of a modern employing organisation. In future, all recruits to the work-force should be appointed with due regard to equal opportunities, and the ethos of 'learning for life' should be visible through continuing professional development. Quality career guidance should also be available for all employees and at all training levels.

The career structure in medicine has been perceived as rigid, with the expectation of frequent moves in the early years, long hours and usually full-time working. There is also a perception that those who could operate the system known as patronage made greater progress than others.[2] Thus a more equitable process of appointing doctors to training programmes is timely, and the new opportunities described within the *Green Guide* should facilitate a more flexible approach to training and lead to a new era of flexible working patterns within the NHS.

In the Trent Region we have elected to appoint doctors to general practice training through selection centres which will assess each candidate's fitness for purpose (i.e. general practice training) before offering them training programmes that will ensure that they emerge fit for general practice. These selection centres are based on the existing assessment centre methodology, which is widely used by major employers across the UK.

Assessment centres are evaluation processes, usually consisting of a day of different job-related exercises which are intended to simulate the major components of the skills and abilities underlying the target job role.[3] Exercises typically include group exercises (e.g. where candidates work together to solve a problem), competency-based interviews, role-play simulation, psychometric ability tests and in-tray exercises (where candidates are asked to respond to messages, memos and other information). The different exercises are observed and assessed by trained assessors on various job-related competencies. Some of these may include communication skills, team involvement and problem-solving ability.

The use of assessment centres is widespread and appears to be on the increase in the UK. In a survey, Robertson and Makin[4] (1986) reported that 20% of organisations used assessment centres for managerial recruitment purposes. In 1991, Shackleton and Newell,[5] in a similar survey, found that 60% of the sample were using assessment centres. Current estimates suggest that over 70% of large UK organisations use assessment centres for selection.[6]

A significant body of literature has shown assessment centres to be the best predictors of future job performance. In terms of reliability and criterion-related validity, the evidence is generally very positive, with assessment centres tending to outperform all other selection techniques in both fairness and accuracy.[7] Unlike other selection methods, the assessment centre technique is based on a multi-trait, multi-method principle. By observing candidate performance in different job-related situations, assessment is generally more accurate than it would be in, say, a 30-minute unstructured interview.

There is a great deal of empirical evidence to support this proposition, For example, in a meta-analysis by Gaugler *et al.*[8] which included over 3000 candidates, the mean validity coefficient between candidate assessment centre performance and later job performance was $r = 0.41$. It is noteworthy that higher validities are usually observed when predicting potential rather than actual performance.

Chan[9] found that assessment centre ratings predicted subsequent promotion after controlling for the current supervisory ratings of job performance. This finding indicates that assessment centre ratings may contain information about learning potential and future success over and above the skills and abilities that are assessed in current job performance. Thus individual performance at an assessment centre may give the recruiter invaluable information about the future potential of candidates. Furthermore, there is evidence to suggest that the applicants tend to favour assessment centres over other selection techniques, probably because of the use of work simulations.[10]

Applying the assessment centre method to selection procedures within the NHS is a radical step, but career development centres for doctors have been piloted.[11]

Whilst knowledge and skills (*can do*) are fundamental to accurate diagnosis and treatment, the values and attitudes (*will do*) exhibited by doctors are key to successful clinical practice. Part of the problem with attitudinal progress may be the heavily 'science'-loaded curriculum at medical schools. Recently, the humanities component of medicine has been expanded, and a greater focus on this area should help to develop the behavioural competencies that are needed by the successful practitioner. These competencies have been described[12] and incorporated into the person specification and assessment exercises used for the Trent Region selection centres.

The new national system for recruitment to general practice training programmes

The Directors of Postgraduate General Practice Education have developed new appointment systems for general practice training programmes. The details of each deanery's selection process will differ slightly, but they are all based on common principles. It is anticipated that the processes will evolve over the next two years. The vision is for all of the deaneries to move gradually towards a common system, perhaps similar to the UCAS process.

The key features will include a biannual national advertisement for all of the English regions or deaneries and the armed forces. The advertisement will describe the training opportunities that are available to doctors who wish to prepare for a career in general practice. It is hoped that the other UK countries will join the advertising and recruitment programme in 2001.

The advertisements will be placed in the *British Medical Journal* and on a number of appropriate websites. They will detail contact points for applications to join a GP training programme, as well as the range of training opportunities available within each region. Both vocational training schemes and free-standing placements in a training practice will be included in the advertisements. They will also include details of opportunities for those doctors who wish to train flexibly or return to practice.

Vacancies will allow for standard rotations, shortened and extended programmes. There will be allocations of training posts to facilitate the return to general practice of previously 'trained' colleagues, and 'special' training for doctors who require updating or a period of 'targeted' supervision and assessment. There will also be more opportunities for doctors who wish to train flexibly.

Structured applications will be closely linked to a national person specification. Structured references will be requested, including one from the doctor's most recent employer. Medical qualification, full registration with the General Medical Council and satisfactory completion of the pre-registration house year (or its equivalent) should be established prior to application. 'Job offers' will be made subject to a previous criminal convictions inquiry, health check and suitable references.

The competencies expected of the successful general practitioner have been described,[12] and should enable the prospective general practice registrar to answer the following key questions. Is general practice the right career for me? *(I know what I want to achieve)*. Am I the right sort of doctor for general practice? *(I am quite capable of achieving it)*. This echoes the point made by Atkinson and McClelland[3] that it is possible to motivate learners if you place two thoughts (*italicised above*) in their working memory.

Applicants will be expected to list the scheme(s) of their choice in rank order. This may increase the likelihood of appointment within a particular region, if this is desirable. In some deaneries, a multiple-choice question (MCQ) paper testing basic medical knowledge may be set as part of the selection process but not as an initial screening procedure. The behavioural competencies expected of general practitioners will be assessed partially from applications but more thoroughly at interview.

Short-listing will be undertaken by a panel which will normally consist of general practitioners, hospital consultants and administrators. Lay members representing users and carers will increasingly be involved in the selection processes.

In the Trent region, selection centres will involve candidates attending for a full day of assessment exercises and interviews. Prospective general practice registrars will have the opportunity to demonstrate that they have reached a point in their professional development which confirms that they are capable of attaining, within a three-year training period, the standards required for independent general practice. The final ranking of candidates will take place after interviews have been completed. A matching process will ensure that the highest-ranked candidates are offered placements in line with their own previously expressed preferences. Feedback will be available to enhance appropriate training for successful candidates and to support unsuccessful candidates.

In other deaneries and regions the selection processes will differ from the Trent model, but they are all firmly rooted in the same principles.

Employment contracts and educational agreements will be exchanged once posts have been agreed. Placements in appropriate general practice training posts will be determined 'locally'. Course organisers will have a key role, and in some regions 'matching schemes' similar to those used in the placement of pre-registration house officers are planned. Trainers and the prospective registrars will continue to have the ability to say no, and there will be no coercion in the placement of doctors into training practices.

Flexibility to move between vocational training schemes will depend on the availability of placements, funding, satisfactory performance of the doctor in previous posts, and the doctor's personal circumstances. The movement of doctors between deaneries will be facilitated by the DsPGPE and co-ordinated nationally.

These changes will contribute to a more equitable, appropriate and fulfilling training system for general practice. Equal opportunities, flexibility and even higher quality educational opportunities will replace the days of multiple applications, several interviews and inappropriate training for the next generation of general practitioners.

References

1 Department of Health (2000) *The GP Registrar Scheme – Vocational Training for General Medical Practice – The UK Green Guide*. Department of Health, London.

2 Allen I, Brown P and Hughes P (eds) (1997) *Choosing Tomorrow's Doctors*. Policy Studies Institute, London.

3 Woodruffe C (2000) *Development and Assessment Centres: Identifying and Assessing Competence* (3e). IPD, London.

4 Robertson I and Makin P (1986) Management selection in Britain: a survey and critique. *J Occup Psychol.* **59**: 45–57.

5 Shackleton V and Newell S (1991) Management selection: a comparative survey of methods used in top British and French companies. *J Occup Psychol.* **64**: 23–36.

6 Shackleton V and Newell S (1997) International selection and assessment. In: N Anderson and P Herriot (eds) *International Handbook of Selection and Assessment*. John Wiley & Sons, Chichester.

7 Schmidt N and Chan D (1998) *Personnel Selection: a Theoretical Approach*. Sage, London.

8 Gaugler B, Rosenthal D, Thornton G and Bentson C (1987) Meta-analysis of assessment centre validity. *J Appl Psychol.* **75**: 698–709.

9 Chan D (1996) Criterion and construct validation of an assessment centre. *J Occup Organis Psychol.* **69**: 167–81.

10 Iles P and Robertson I (1997) The impact of personnel selection procedures on candidates. In: N Anderson and P Herriot (eds) *International Handbook of Selection and Assessment.* John Wiley & Sons, Chichester.

11 Kisely S (1998) Career development centres for doctors. *BMJ.* **316**.

12 Ferguson E, Patterson F, Lane P *et al.* (2000) Behavioural competencies of general practitioners. *Br J Gen Pract.* **50**: 188–93.

12

Educating the GP in a primary care-led NHS: what are the problems with training in hospitals?

Christopher Hand and Anne McKee

Introduction

The main aim of this chapter is to discuss the contribution that hospitals can make to the training of future general practitioners (GPs). This discussion takes place in rapidly changing political and medical environments. In the past decade, reform of the NHS has reshaped the role of the GP and the organisational structure within which general medical services are delivered. The recent announcement of extra financial investment in the National Health Service (NHS) and the need for more doctors means that further change is inevitable. Medical educationalists will be heavily involved in the process of interpreting and delivering those changes. As the role of the GP and the context of care continue to evolve within the unfolding Labour modernisation agenda, a reconsideration of the training for the GP seems appropriate, if not imperative. The obvious question to ask is the following one. *Why should future GPs spend two years in hospital and only one in general practice, when the latter is the context in which they will deliver care?*

The opportunity to change training is here

The transfer of funding to the Medical and Dental Education Levy (MADEL) has created an opportunity for GPs to review the whole process of vocational training.[1] The chairman of the Royal College of General Practitioners (RCGP),

Professor Mike Pringle, has recently gone on record as saying that senior house officer (SHO) posts need to be reformed.[2] This position reflects a widely held belief among GP educationalists that much of hospital training serves the needs of providing a hospital service and not the needs of professional preparation for general practice. Is this a valid view, or are we in danger of throwing the baby out with the bath water? As educationalists we need to identify what GPs learn from their hospital training posts and how much of this is useful for the professional challenges that they will face in general practice.

Before embarking on widespread reform of hospital training for GP SHOs, it would seem sensible to explore the views of the profession as a whole. We also need to know the answers to some basic questions.

- What is it that a GP does that only a GP can do?
- How might they best learn what they need to know and be able to do?
- Where might they best learn it?

The historical context

In 1966, the RCGP proposed four years of training for general practice after registration. However, the final recommendation of the Todd Report was even more generous and recommended five years' training. When the NHS (Vocational Training) Regulations were finally issued in 1979 they stipulated only three years' training. This has been described as a compromise by the RCGP,[3] but in fact our discipline was badly let down. What is worse, this created a three-year structure of vocational training that was held in place by legislative authority. The structure could only be changed by further legislation – a strait-jacket that would stifle the ability of training to adapt to changing needs and circumstances for the rest of the century.

Theoretically, the middle year of training could be taken in general practice but the money to fund it was never available. Most vocational training schemes therefore provided six-month rotations over two years in first-list posts.[4] One of the educational assumptions of early schemes was the importance of general medicine, but the advance of specialisation has restructured this discipline into a complex framework of minor specialities.

In 1994, the RCGP highlighted the need for more training time in general practice to take account of the changes in GPs' work following the introduction of the New Contract. The College recommended an equal split of 18 months in hospital and 18 months in general practice. The Educational Incentive Programme (LIZEI) which provided additional funding made this possible in London. Some innovative schemes have already altered the balance between hospital and general practice training,[5] encouraged the development of new hospital posts[6] and also extended the training to four years.[7]

The political and social context

Over the past 10 years the medical profession has increasingly been made publicly accountable. Currently the medical profession is subject to media scrutiny as several high-profile cases dominate the news. The role of the General Medical Council (GMC) has been called into question by the profession itself with a vote of no confidence, and the future of professional self-regulation appears to be under threat.

With the rise of accountability came the demands of consumerism. The consumerist approach to medicine promised quick and convenient access to medical care regardless of the seriousness of the condition. The appearance of walk-in centres and NHS Direct is a political response to social pressure. That social pressure is to protect the vision of a service that is available at the point of need. Walk-in centres and NHS Direct offer an illusion of matching demand for medical services with supply. Their introduction, following a period during which a structure for the systematic rationing of services has been introduced, reflects an enduring problem, namely how to offer all that medical care is capable of while at the same time containing the costs.

The changing medical context

Changes to the organisational structure of the NHS have stimulated other changes to the role and workload of the GP. As managerial responsibilities increased and the profession perceived that the working day was becoming longer and more intense, GPs began to develop ways of prioritising their clinical workload and engaging with the challenge to plan and deliver local care. These included delegating clinical work to nurses, and creating out-of-hours co-operatives. The emerging issue appears to be what type of service it is appropriate and reasonable to expect a GP to offer.

Primary care groups (PCGs) and primary care trusts (PCTs) look set to change the face of general practice even more than the introduction of the New Contract in 1990. The prospect of a salaried service for GPs looks highly likely, despite the resistance of the British Medical Association's General Practice Committee. Although management skills are needed to run practices and PCG/PCT boards, how much time GPs will spend on management rather than medicine remains to be seen. However, there is no doubt that more time will be spent on education, given the introduction of revalidation, but the effects of this on service provision have not been adequately thought through.

Secondary care has not escaped change either. The radical restructuring of specialist training[8] and the reduction of junior doctors' hours are having profound effects on the hospital service. Although these two developments cannot be held entirely to blame for lengthening waiting-lists and bed crises, they have not helped. It is not surprising that care is being shifted from secondary to primary care, and that intermediate care is being heralded as a possible solution to the problem of caring for an older population.

What does the literature tell us?

Is this just a problem for GPs?

SHO posts have been criticised for many years. This criticism has extended to both SHO training in general[9–11] and general practice training in particular.[12–17] The problems are not related to any one speciality[18–20] or any one region.[18,21–24] In fact, it is a national problem affecting the UK as a whole,[15] Scotland[25,26] and Ireland,[27] and it is also an international problem.[28]

Is it all bad?

Most of the published evidence emphasises the negative aspects of hospital training. This is not entirely surprising given that in 1999 less than 5% of all posts that were approved for GP training were graded as excellent, despite the fact that nearly half of them were only given conditional approval (Hospital Recognition Committee of the RCGP, personal communication, 2000). Suggestions have been made as to how the training in hospital might be improved[29] and made more relevant to GPs.[30–32] However, there are some signs that SHO training may be improving,[33,34] but only limited evidence that this applies to GP training posts.[35,36] Yet considerable changes to junior hospital posts can be achieved if there is the will to do this.[37]

What are the problems?

The following main problems were identified from the Joint Hospital Visits of the RCGP with other Royal Colleges:

- inadequate induction
- lack of educational objectives
- teaching of little relevance to general practice
- poor clinical support
- lack of personal feedback
- lack of protected teaching time

- lack of study leave and personal study time
- difficulty in attending half-day release for GPs
- poor domestic arrangements
- lack of involvement in audit
- stressful jobs.

All of these issues have been identified in the published literature and summarised by McEvoy.[31] They reflect the many tensions that exist between education and service. However, not all of the issues are insoluble, and some of them could be addressed relatively easily. For instance, educational object-ives are published jointly by the RCGP and other specialist Royal Colleges,[38] although their use is not universal. More recently, Royal Colleges have started to provide structured curricula and log books for SHOs. At present there is no national logbook for the hospital component of GP training, although some regions have introduced them (Bahrami, personal communication, 2000).

Why has it taken so long for things to change?

Unfortunately, SHO training has had to take a back seat while changes to specialist registrar training[8] and improvements to pre-registration training[39] have been introduced. The GMC has only recently focused its attention on SHO training,[40] and so it is not entirely surprising that SHOs have been described as the 'lost tribes'.[11]

Despite these factors, there still appears to be a resistance by hospitals to adapt to educational change for SHOs. Part of the problem is the difference in perception between those who do the training and those who receive it.[10,41] Another factor is the enduring belief of consultants that an apprenticeship experience is the most powerful contribution to training.[42] Shortage of time, both for consultants and for junior doctors, is a further issue. There is a feeling that partial shifts, which are increasingly being used to cope with the reduction in junior doctors' hours, have detrimental effects on education and training.[43] Lack of educational training has also been blamed,[42] but this problem is being addressed by teaching the teachers to teach programmes.[44]

Why do we need more evidence?

While preparing to write a chapter on hospital training for the third edition of *The GP Training Handbook*,[45] one of us (CH) contacted all of the regions in the UK to obtain information about the hospital component of their vocational training schemes. It soon became apparent that there was a diversity of opinion in relation to both the necessity for GPs to train in hospital and also the quality of the hospital training. The variation in quality is consistent with the joint hospital visiting reports received by the RCGP Hospital Recognition Committee and the highly critical evidence from the literature.

Most of the published research has been conducted using quantitative surveys at a regional level. There is much less qualitative work.[10,16,23] Surveys of GP registrars/trainees, trainers and course organisers are common,[22,15,46] but the voice of hospital consultants is rarely heard.[16,42] Given the importance of the relationship between GPs and consultants in hospitals where significant improvements have taken place,[35,37,47] this appears to be a major omission.

What is EDGE?

Educating the General Practitioner in a Primary Care-Led NHS (EDGE) is a qualitative study of current vocational training provision within the East Anglian Deanery, involving both medical and academic educationalists. The project team comes from the Schools of Education and Professional Development and Health Policy and Practice at the University of East Anglia. The project is investigating the changing role of the GP, the changing contexts of practice, the current training provision in both hospital and general practice, and how that provision is valued by trainers and registrars. A series of interviews and focus groups is being held with GP educationalists, GP and consultant teachers, GP registrars and patients. The participants come from four GP vocational training schemes selected to represent contrasting training environments. A critical part of the study is to explore the role of hospitals in training for general practice. Some of the emerging themes from this qualitative study will be used to highlight the issues that are now facing us.

Despite receiving funding from the Eastern NHS Executive Research and Development Subcommittee, the methodology continues to be viewed with suspicion by local research ethics committees and consultants. Having eventually secured access to the four sites (some six months into the project), we are still improving access within hospitals.

The research is addressing the following questions.

Interpreting requirements in the changing context of primary care

- What recent changes have taken place in the formal requirements for general practice?
- How do general practitioners interpret these requirements in their particular primary care context?
- How is the job changing? What are the major changes that general practitioners experience in the practice context, and how do they perceive

them to impinge on their work (e.g. as demands, pressures, constraints, dilemmas, freedoms and opportunities)?
- How do the external requirements interact with the primary care context to shape the work of general practitioners?

Hospital training and general practice

- Within the specialist areas that are most relevant to GP training, how do hospital consultants understand the changing demands on general practitioners?
- Do hospital consultants perceive hospital training within their speciality to be responsive to both the formal requirements for primary care and the changing demands that are experienced in the general practice context? If so, how? Are there specific training policies within their speciality?

Hospital training and professional learning

- What do general practitioners think that they learned from their hospital training?
  (i) Things that they were intended to learn formally and informally.
  (ii) Things that they learned as unintended side-effects.
- Which of the following types of hospital-based learning do general practitioners perceive themselves to have used and applied in a sustainable form within their professional work?
  (i) Medical knowledge (both substantive and procedural).
  (ii) Interpersonal skills in relation to patients and/or colleagues/partners.
  (iii) Capacity for clinical judgement.
- What do general practitioners perceive themselves to have learned from their specialist hospital training that it would have been difficult or impossible for them to have learned solely within the general practice context?
- What do hospital consultants understand to be the knowledge and skills that general practitioners can best learn in the context of hospital training?

The organisation of professional preparation for general practitioners

- How do organisational structures interact with the curriculum structures to shape the learning experiences of GP trainees?
- How, in the perception of general practitioners, might preparation for general practice be effectively and appropriately organised?

What issues are emerging?

Perceptions of hospital training include the following.

Course organisers

Course organisers shared the reservations of GP trainers that much of the hospital training experience was inappropriate. Despite this they also claimed that GP SHOs developed the following knowledge and skills from their hospital posts:

• knowing and managing common presenting conditions and emergencies
• gaining insight into the relevance of hospital work and its organisation
• learning when hospital referral is appropriate
• informing patients about what will happen to them in hospital
• developing confidence through knowledge and experience
• learning essential aspects of specialities to make them a safer and better GP.

Exploring the apparent contradiction in these views, we asked what was inappropriate about the training, and whether there was anything worth preserving. Training was felt to be inappropriate in two ways. First, it prioritised the need to provide a medical service, and secondly, it often failed to focus on what was relevant and important for future GPs. Dissatisfaction with current hospital training appeared to lie with both the belief and the experience that the potential of hospital training would not be realised within the current framework and culture of hospital training.

We asked what would improve hospital training. The list identified both service contexts where GP SHOs would be most likely to encounter clinical activity appropriate to their future professional needs, and the adoption of methods and values of vocational training. The list of suggested improvements included the following:

• more out-patient and clinic work
• better organised teaching relevant to primary care
• more small group/interactive teaching
• less humiliation
• less ward-round teaching
• more communication skills teaching.

Is dissatisfaction with hospital training due to the need for specialist training or to frustration with the constraints under which hospital training is provided?

GP trainers

The views of GP trainers were similar to those of course organisers. One asserted that hospital training 'feels like a rite of passage, something to be endured rather than valued.' During a focus group session with GP trainees, course organisers and GP trainers, one trainer commented that 'we are all singing out of the same hymn-book', emphasising the commonality and consensus of the group when critiquing hospital training.

Once more, running parallel to the critique of hospital training were a number of claims of significant benefits. These included the following:

- developing confidence and maturity
- managing common conditions
- learning to work as part of a team
- learning to be confident in managing and diagnosing conditions in a particular speciality
- following through diseases and thus knowing their natural history
- seeing many common problems that are relevant to general practice
- studying for examinations (e.g. Diploma in Child Health)
- gaining a breadth of clinical experience
- dealing with emergencies and recognising seriously ill patients
- emergency life support training (many value Accident and Emergency experience)
- learning when hospital referral is appropriate
- informing patients about what will happen to them in hospital.

This list raises some other questions, namely how many of these learning outcomes and opportunities are available only through hospital training, and what it is that hospital training does that only hospital training can do.

GP registrars

While exploring the GP SHO experience of hospital training we encountered different notions of what appropriate training entailed. For many, appropriate training was about the acquisition of knowledge. Being prepared for general practice was about knowing enough from a range of specialities for them to know what to do when in practice. Some of those in hospital complained of erratic informal teaching from specialist registrars, and only occasional tutorials with consultants. Those in the final year of training still talked about the importance of knowing enough, but this was tempered by the sense that being prepared for practice included more than having sufficient knowledge.

Philosophically the notion of appropriate training is contentious, particularly if decisions have to be made about whose view counts and why. An emerging issue in our research is that GP trainers and course organisers have different ideas about what is an appropriate training for general practice for many GP SHOs. Trainers appear to emphasise the importance of GP SHOs being able to survive a lifetime in practice. In contrast, many SHOs want to get through summative assessment and begin their career as a GP. Trainers bring to their training a complex understanding of the realities and challenges of the job. GP SHOs bring the perspective of novices who tend to be more closely focused on the basics of what it takes to do the job. We are exploring this difference by asking the following questions.

- What is it that a GP needs to know and to be able to do?
- How much of that is it feasible and necessary to learn within vocational training?

It is perhaps easy to underestimate the gap between an experienced GP and a novice one. To the experienced GP, their identity as a GP and the culture of general practice have become integral parts of their professional self. To the trainee GP, both their identity as a GP and the culture of general practice are new. Their professional selves and culture are still drawing upon the experiences of hospital medicine. It seems that one of the aspects of hospital training which they value is belonging to a group of junior doctors – having colleagues and peers to talk to, to socialise with and to learn from. For some, general practice can be a more isolating experience. We are beginning to explore how GP SHOs fit into the group of hospital SHOs, what membership implies, and what values they accept or challenge. With a foot in two professional cultures, one of these being hospital medicine and the other general practice, the GP SHO is exposed to different knowledge bases, models of care, attitudes to patients, power structures and judges. We are exploring the impact of this on what they learn, how they learn it, and their view of general practice.

Consultants

Interviews with consultants help to illuminate the changing service and learning environment within hospitals. At this stage of the study, three themes appear to characterise those changes, namely generationalisation, resources issues and the consultant professional culture and its implications for teaching.

Generationalisation

Nearly all of the consultants interviewed to date have talked about differences between pre- and post-Calman consultants. (There are very few consultants trained completely within the Calman structure, but there appear to be a reasonable number of those whose final stages of training have been accelerated.) Both sides of the generation gap pointed to differences in the other. Older consultants seem to feel that their younger colleagues do not have the knowledge, skills and attitudes of those who were trained pre-Calman. They suggest that the shorter period of training has meant that recently qualified consultants have not had the breadth of clinical experience of their predecessors. Younger consultants have found that older consultants can be resistant to change. That resistance may be about protecting long-standing practice rather than adopting new approaches or protecting resources. Most change implies finance.

We are also finding that specialities are resourced at different levels and have their own professional values with regard to multiprofessional and team-based care.

Resource issues

The Calman reforms have made necessary the formalisation of training and have shortened the training period. In most specialities there is a feeling that the new educational demands have not been backed up by additional resources. The two-hour teaching round envisaged by Calman does not happen.

Another resource issue concerns the role of nurses. Consultants identified differences in the care of patients and the management of wards following changes in the professional roles and training of nurses. Some consultants experience this as a reduction in nursing cover (because nurses are not available to look after patients and take note of medical management plans). This has had an effect on ward-based education: 'You wander into the ward and you try and find the patient, who is in the bath, and the nurse who is looking after her says "I'm on the green team today, but I'm with Mrs Smith at the moment" '.[48]

This contrasts with the good old days when the wards were closed to visitors, registrars followed the consultant round the ward, and the patients were in bed ready for examination. Others have described the current management of wards as 'chaos'.

In the accounts of consultants new and old, there is a sense of fragmentation. They talk about problems of continuity resulting from SHOs who are in a department for short periods, SHOs who accept posts but do not come or else leave early, and the need to use locums. This has implications for the provision of both service and training. Consultants argue that it is difficult to provide coherent training, and there is a drift towards training as a series of isolated events.

There appear to be significant differences across specialities. In some specialities registrars are supernumerary, whilst in others they are integral to the provision of the service.

Consultant professional culture and its implications for teaching

Many career clinicians do not perceive a training role to be part of their chosen career structure, whilst other consultants take a special interest in the training needs of GP SHOs. Consultant attitudes towards training are increasingly important as opportunities to learn from the job change. Ward rounds no longer appear to offer the opportunities for teaching that they once did. Shorter working hours have undermined the basic principle of training by assimilation. It seems that Calmanisation has shifted medical training towards a more formal and programme-based structure. It appears that log books provide a curriculum – in theory if not in practice. In making the most of the learning environment, much depends on the maturity and personality of the registrar. Does 'self-directed' mean 'do-it-yourself'?

If it does, that is not the case across all specialities. It seems that in psychiatry the hidden curriculum is particularly useful to the GP SHO, with its emphasis on developing coping mechanisms, learning about the self and understanding human behaviour.

Apart from the fragmentation already described, the context of hospital medicine has become busier. There are many reasons for this. Some are due to the advance of medical knowledge and techniques making a greater range of interventions possible, while others are resource issues, particularly the need for more doctors and shorter working hours. New rotas make continuity of care difficult, so consultants stay behind and provide it. One consultant said 'As a junior doctor I worked hard so that the consultant could play golf. As a consultant I now work hard so that junior doctors can play golf.'

Such busyness creates a tension between the possible and the desirable. Many consultants told us that they took education seriously but they had real constraints within which to operate.

Some had reservations about the discipline of general practice and, by implication, training for it. 'I can't keep up in my field, how do GPs manage?' asked one consultant, although the question recurred across interviews. As hospital medicine becomes more specialised, the possibility of a generalist being up-to-date was questioned. 'You get some crazy referrals ... we should take away GP referral capacity and give it to physiotherapists', one consultant suggested. Other consultants doubted either the value of general practice or the quality of the practitioners within it. One suggested that general practice as a discipline had no future. What effects does this have on how GP SHOs are valued or treated?

Conclusions

The service and learning environments of general practice and hospitals are changing radically and rapidly. In response to College demands for reform, we have explored the context of change and focused on perceptions and experiences of training in hospital. The demands of service have transformed and are transforming the experience of those who work there. Consultants indicate that, increasingly, service and training needs pull in diverging directions. As specialities form subspecialities, the race for expert status changes. Straddling both worlds, the GP SHOs live within two cultures which appear to have different views about what knowledge is and how one acquires it. GP trainers have been concerned that their discipline is not valued by hospital doctors. We now find that some consultants doubt that the discipline has a future. In the next phase of our research we shall be observing teaching in hospitals in order both to verify the perceptions of those interviewed and to investigate further what SHOs learn when in hospital.

Acknowledgements

We thank the consultants, GP trainers, VTS course organisers and GP registrars who have given so freely of their time. Thanks also to our colleagues in EDGE: Professor John Elliott, Dr Rob Walker, Mrs Jill Schostak and Ms Christine Spooner. NHS Eastern Executive Research and Development Subcommittee funded this study.

References

1   Field S, Allen K, Jackson N *et al.* (2000) Vocational training: the dawn of a new era? *Educ Gen Pract.* **11**: 3–8.

2   Beecham L (2000) Medicopolitical digest. *BMJ.* **320**: 878.

3   Royal College of General Practitioners (1994) *Education and Training for General Practice. Policy Statement 3.* Royal College of General Practitioners, London.

4   Joint Committee on Postgraduate Training for General Practice (1995) *Posts in Hospital and Public Health Medicine: General Guidance.* JCPTGP, London.

5   Savage R, Kiernan E and Reuben LA (1996) Registrar training for general practice: a pilot study of 18 months of hospital posts and 18 months in general practice. *Educ Gen Pract.* **7**: 191–8.

6   Savage R, Torry R, Vaughan C and Horner B (1997) Vocational training for general practice: course organiser controlled funding to construct innovative SHO posts. *Educ Gen Pract.* **8**: 280–7.

7   Toon PD, Jackson N, Pietroni PC *et al.* (1999) Extended GP registrarships: the LIZEI experiment. *Educ Gen Pract.* **10**: 437–41.

8   Department of Health (1993) *Hospital Doctors: Training for the Future. The Report of the Working Group on Specialist Medical Training (Calman Report)*. Department of Health, London.

9   COPMeD (1987) *The Problems of the Senior House Officer*. COPMeD, London.

10   Grant J, Marsden P and King RC (1989) Senior house officers and their training. I. Personal characteristics and professional circumstances. II. Perceptions of service and training. *BMJ.* **299**: 1263–8.

11   Dillner L (1993) Senior house officers: the lost tribes. *BMJ.* **307**: 1549–51.

12   Ronalds C, Douglas A, Gray DP *et al.* (1981) *Fourth National Trainee Conference. Report, Recommendations and Questionnaire*. Occasional Paper 18. Royal College of General Practitioners, London.

13   Evans S (1987) Hospital component of vocational training. *J Assoc Course Organisers.* **3**: 46.

14   Styles WMcN (1990) General practice training in the hospital. *Br J Gen Pract.* **40**: 401–2.

15   Crawley HS and Levin JB (1990) Training for general practice: a national survey. *BMJ.* **300**: 911–15.

16   Kearley K (1990) An evaluation of the hospital component of general practice vocational training. *Br J Gen Pract.* **40**: 409–14.

17   Hand CH and Adams M (1998) The development and reliability of the Royal College of General Practitioners questionnaire for measuring senior house officers' satisfaction with their hospital training. *Br J Gen Pract.* **48**: 1399–403.

18   Polnay L and Pringle M (1989) General practitioner training in paediatrics in the Trent region. *BMJ.* **298**: 1434–6.

19   Smith LFP (1991) GP trainees' views on hospital obstetric vocational training. *BMJ.* **303**: 1147–52.

20   Ogg EC, Pugh R and Murray TS (1997) Scottish general practice registrars: their views on psychotherapy training. *Br J Gen Pract.* **47**: 723–5.

21   Reeve H and Bowman A (1989) Hospital training for general practice: views of trainees in the North Western region. *BMJ.* **298**: 1432–4.

22   Little P (1994) What do Wessex general practitioners think about the structure of hospital vocational training? *BMJ.* **308**: 1337–9.

23   Torry R (1996) The training needs of hospital general practice registrars in SE Thames. *Educ Gen Pract.* **7**: 280–7.

24   Bunch GA, Bahrami J and MacDonald R (1997) Training in the SHO grade. *Br J Hosp Med.* **57**: 565–8.

25   Kelly DR and Murray TS (1991) Twenty years of vocational training in the west of Scotland. *BMJ.* **302**: 28–30.

26   Kelly D and Murray TS (1997) An assessment of hospital training for general practice in Scotland. *Educ Gen Pract.* **8**: 220–6.

27   Murphy M (1995) The hospital component of general practice vocational training: persistent preventable problems. *Educ Gen Pract.* **6**: 19–29.

28   Rotem A, Godwin P and Du J (1993) *Review of the Hospital Learning Environment for the Family Medicine Programme.* School of Medical Education, University of New South Wales, Sydney, pp. 1–126.

29   Baker M (1993) Enhancing the educational content of SHO posts. *BMJ.* **306**: 808–9.

30   Murphy M (1995) The hospital component of general practice vocational training: persistent preventable problems. *Educ Gen Pract.* **6**: 19–29.

31   McEvoy P (1998) *Educating the Future GP. The Course Organisers' Handbook* (2e) Radcliffe Medical Press, Oxford.

32   Hand CH (1999) Hospital training. In: MS Hall, D Dwyer and A Lewis (eds) *The GP Training Handbook* (3e). Blackwell Science, Oxford.

33   Paice E, West G, Cooper R, Orton V and Scotland A (1997) Senior house officer training: is it getting better? *BMJ.* **314**: 719–20.

34   Paice E, Aitken M, Cowan G and Heard S (2000) Trainee satisfaction before and after the Calman reforms of specialist training: questionnaire survey. *BMJ.* **320**: 832–6.

35   Rickenbach M, Dunleavy J, Little P and Mullee M (1997) Impact of existing peer review visits needs to be increased. *BMJ.* **314**: 1829–30.

36   Hand CH (2000) Evaluating satisfaction with hospital training for general practice: a comparison of two surveys in East Anglia for the JCPTGP using the RCGP SHO questionnaire. *Educ Gen Pract.* **11**: 385–90.

37   Moore JK, Neithercut WD, Mellors AS *et al.* (1994) Making the new deal for junior doctors happen. *BMJ.* **308**: 1553–5.

38   Royal College of General Practitioners (1997) *The Quality of Hospital-Based Education for General Practice.* Royal College of General Practitioners, London.

39   General Medical Council (1997) *The New Doctor.* General Medical Council, London.

40   General Medical Council (1998) *The Early Years: Recommendations on Senior House Officer Training.* General Medical Council, London.

41   Baker M and Sprackling PD (1994) The educational component of senior house officer posts: differences in the perceptions of consultants and junior doctors. *Postgrad Med J.* **70**: 198–202.

42   Wilson DH (1993) Education and training of pre-registration house officers: the consultants' viewpoint. *BMJ.* **306**: 194–6.

43   Mather HM and Connor H (2000) Coping with pressures in acute medicine – the second RCP consultant questionnaire survey. *J R Coll Physicians Lond.* **34**: 371–3.

44   Wall D (1999) Twelve tips on teaching the consultant teachers to teach. *Med Teacher.* **21**: 387–92.

45 Hall MS, Dwyer D and Lewis A (eds) (1999) *The GP Training Handbook* (3e). Blackwell Science, Oxford.

46 Styles WMcN, Grant J, Golombok S *et al.* (1993) The hospital component of vocational training for general practice: the views of course organisers. *Postgrad Educ Gen Pract.* **4**: 203–8.

47 Tait I (1987) Agreed educational objectives for the hospital period of vocational training. *J Assoc Course Organisers.* **2**: 179–82.

48 Schostak JF, Schostak JR, McKee A and Hand CH (1999) *A Six-Month Study of Junior Doctor Learning Experiences.* Centre for Applied Research in Education (CARE), School of Education and Professional Development, University of East Anglia, Norwich.

13

A way forward: a description of the process and outcomes of a review of vocational training in South Thames East

Ian McLean

This process was carried out in order to advance the development of the support of vocational training in this deanery, questioning what we *think* we do now and what we *think* we ought to do in the future.

Reasons for conducting the review

Although it is clear that, in general terms, vocational training for general practice has not changed much since its inception, significant changes are now about to take place.[1,2] We need to acknowledge and respond to the new concepts of work-force planning and fitness for purpose, stimulated by the development of Local Work-force Planning Groups and the transfer of the funding of the process of vocational training to the deaneries (known as the MADEL transfer).

It is also clear that the aims of training are not now necessarily compatible with those of the ever-changing NHS, and that the service requirements of the NHS, rarely influence the training agenda.[3]

There are now defined priorities for 2000.[4] These include the enhanced management of the general practice element and the enhanced educational role of hospital placements. There is a need to improve study leave arrangements, and there also needs to be a planned educational programme for both the hospital and general practice components. Study leave needs to be planned and enhanced. It has therefore been suggested that the demands of training for general practice now necessitate an increase in the length of time that is spent in the general practice component.

Thus, whilst we realised that there is a strong move to increase the total time spent in vocational training, there is also scope for improvement within the current structures, and we decided that this should be the focus of our review.

Review process

Trainers and course organisers were informed of the proposed process by letter, and were invited to express an interest in being involved. To support them, locum fees were paid for attendance at the working parties. Three small working parties were organised, each meeting on three occasions for about three hours, and notes were written up, circulated and developed sequentially.

The group that was looking at course organising consisted of two course organisers, a trainer and a registrar. The group that was looking at training issues consisted of two trainers, a course organiser and a GP registrar. The group that was looking at issues related to trainer selection committees and processes consisted of the chairs of the three Regional Patch Trainer Selection Committees and of the Postgraduate Education Board. Each group was facilitated and supported by a GP associate adviser and a continuing professional development (CPD) associate adviser.

General aims

There were three main objectives. Starting with the existing job descriptions for trainers and course organisers, the first aim was to produce a new job description for course organisers and for trainers that would reflect the responsibilities inherent in the job today. This would also recognise the ways in which training for trainers and continuing skills enhancement could be developed.

The second aim was that the review should describe ways in which vocational training could be drawn closer to the other areas of continuing general practice education.

Finally, it should suggest more appropriate ways in which the trainer selection process could be conducted.

Thus the areas of focus for the working parties included the following:

- job description
- training and career path
- skills introduction and enhancement
- appraisal
- continuing professional development.

Reviewing the present situation

The working groups looked at the present job descriptions and considered the following questions.

- What is now the status and role of GP educators?
- With reference to the present system of course organisers and GP tutors, what are the routes for getting there?
- Is there any equality?
- Do course organisers have greater perceived 'status' than GP tutors?
- There may be a perceived path leading from GP to trainer, to course organiser, to possible associate dean/director, to possible dean/director. Is this really how it should be?
- Where in this route do GP tutors come in?
- How are these roles perceived from viewpoints outside the training world?
- How do course organisers and GP tutors relate to one another generally?

The conclusions that the working parties reached included the sense that at present there is inadequate support for individuals to develop educational skills and roles.[5] Certainly there is no formal educational career path that is appropriately validated. There is inadequate support and induction for individuals who decide to take on these roles, and there are difficulties related to continuity and succession. These include the impression that the jobs of course organisers, for example, have a 'cosiness' about them that may be engendered by the normally open-ended contract (i.e. although the contract runs for three years, if the incumbent wishes to continue there is rarely a challenge to this). On the other hand, the inertia of this situation may give rise to difficulties in stimulating local interest in a replacement when the time comes. It also makes it more difficult to introduce new models of vocational training when these become appropriate.

Course organisers and trainers recognised the need for more continuing support. This would include both the infrastructure supporting the administration (e.g. by having a well-organised central office structure that could respond to questions from trainers and course organisers quickly and efficiently), and a continuing process of skills development.

General outcomes and ideas

There was a strong sense of the need for development of a deanery education role (or roles) within a pool or team that was locally based (local educational teams). These should include GPs, but should not be solely composed of them.

These teams should have an active and formal role in relation to the primary/ secondary care education interface.

There must be a clear relationship with primary care groups or trusts, especially with regard to revalidation and continuing professional development. There should be recognition of an educator career path in general practice, which is properly paid and supported relative to the clinical practice role, and having equal status with that role.

There should be processes to ensure that individuals are formally trained for these roles (e.g. ability to work with and in groups, or dealing with SHO selection/continuing educational needs, etc.). This would enhance the move towards increased continuity and co-ordination of education, with the loss of the culture of fragmentation and splitting that is a feature at present.

Specific development issues for VTS course organisers

These would need to include areas such as facilitation skills, group management skills and the ability to perform effective learning needs assessments for GP registrars, both in hospital posts and in general practice. It would also be necessary to be able to review processes of managing the regular educational activity and development of the skills, in order to manage the issues that arise from these.

The processes for delivering education would need to be enhanced and developed. There should be formal liaison and regular communication with the GP tutors, the (newly forming) primary care tutors and the educational and clinical governance leads of the PCG/PCTs. They should have a formal input to the appraisal of all of the VTS SHOs during their hospital jobs. Finally, perhaps it is time to get rid of the term 'half-day release course', with its connotations of penal escape and its continuing tendency to be translated as 'play school', and to move towards defining the process as what it really is – for example, VTS Group Development Programme (or something similar).

In order to help to increase awareness of development needs for course organisers, there should be an active process of appraisal, enhanced by the present process, which should include feedback. This should come from SHOs and GP registrars, and from the trainer group, and it could also include the use of video recordings of teaching sessions or review processes either with individuals or with the group as a whole.

Specific development issues for VTS trainers

Although it was recognised that trainers will need to play a greater role in the development of a locally enhanced educational process, as described above, the main focus of their skills development will be as educationalists working in a one-to-one relationship.

In order for this to happen, it is important that there should be a well-functioning trainer group.

Here again there was some discussion of terminology. For a long time the term 'trainer workshop' has been used to describe the group as well as its meetings. This term seems to have been widely embraced at the time when it was coming into vogue, probably 20 years ago. Perhaps it is more useful now just to use the term 'trainer group', and to reserve the term 'workshop' for an event when an active process of learning or skills development is planned to take place.

It is clear that different groups were in different stages of development, and to achieve congruity of functioning it would be necessary for further input and support to these. It was strongly felt that there was a need to develop the formation and support of facilitators and mentors within the groups. This process would need to be enhanced by deanery skills training processes, either functioning at a wider level or devolved locally.

Thus not only would individuals benefit from enhancing their own educational skills, but the group could then act as a resource to manage the learning needs that arise from reselection or appraisal for trainers.

The process of appraisal was considered to be in great need of development. At present it only takes place in any formal way at reapproval, and it is thus both infrequent and linked to a summative process. Again it was felt that instituting a process for it to occur formally every year could enhance that appraisal. The process should involve peers, and should allow feedback from the registrar formative assessments. It could thus stimulate the development of a trainer's personal learning portfolio. If they were to appraise colleagues effectively, trainers would need training in appraisal techniques, and this would benefit from the resources of the group.

Within this context the trainer groups would foster skills, act as an information source and provide a venue for structured feedback. They would have an important role in helping individual trainers to construct their personal development programmes, and perhaps in managing that process. By liaising and networking with the course organiser(s), GP and primary care tutors, they would access and share these other resources.

Selection processes for VTS trainers

It was strongly felt that these needed to be improved, not only with regard to the management of the structure of the process, but also to include the issues raised by consideration of trainer development.

It was felt that selection processes for VTS trainers should always be locally based if possible, with peer involvement. The process should always involve assessment rather than just an interview (which should be reserved only for difficult situations), and should assess the trainers' performance according to the job description. This job description should include the necessary skills, and it should also specify the outcome that would be expected in the job. These outcomes would by clarified by, and would also clarify, the appraisal, which should lead to recognition of the learning needs. The job description should also reflect the educational and personal career aspirations of the trainer.

Moving the process on...

These suggestions have a number of implications, particularly in the context of a major change in culture. Strong support will be needed to achieve them, with adequate finance. The gain is that this will generate a new framework for the VTS process in which there will be a sense of local ownership of the education of future GPs by GP educators and trainers, and the VTS group development programme will not be seen as merely the province and responsibility of the course organisers. New job descriptions for both course organisers and trainers have been drafted, reflecting the principles described above.

References

1   Department of Health (1998) *The New NHS: Modern, Dependable*. Department of Health, London.

2   Department of Health (2000) *A Health Service of all the Talents: Developing the NHS Work-force*. Department of Health, London.

3   Bahrami J, Evans A and Belton A (2000) Re-structuring the delivery of vocational training for general practice. *Educ Gen Pract.* **11**: 132–7.

4   Field S, Allen K *et al.* (2000) Vocational training: the dawn of a new era? *Educ Gen Pract.* **11**: 3–8.

5   Stephens C and Woodcock A (1999) What are the learning needs of new GP teachers? *Educ Gen Pract.* **10**: 237–44.

14

GP registrar training: what has lasting value?

Ed Peile

Needs and wants of GP registrars – what is the evidence?

Published surveys of trainees' views on their training year have usually been conducted at the conclusion of training, and none of them have addressed what has added value to lifelong learning in general practice.[1–10] Only when trainees have been working as general practitioners for a considerable length of time are they in a position to provide reflective feedback on which elements of their training have proved the most worthwhile in practice. Vocational training is an expensive process, and we need to look at how can it be improved.

Since the work of Freeman and Byrne in 1976,[11] there have been attempts to look critically at vocational training[12,13] and at continuing medical education.[14] Despite some very erudite analysis,[15–17] much remains elusive about the process of learning and what facilitates the development of excellence in general practitioners.

We know that during vocational training knowledge increases to a peak, which is maintained for the first ten years of postgraduate practice, and which declines thereafter.[18] Although some qualitative research shows that education plays only a relatively small part in influencing doctors' behaviour,[18] there is evidence that vocationally trained general practitioners are 'better' general practitioners in terms of 'performing the tasks of a general practitioner to a level of providing quality care'.[19] This evidence, which was published by Hindmarsh in 1998,[20] was multifaceted, but it could not shed light on the processes that contribute to the improvement.

Obtaining consumers' perceptions – the Aylesbury experiment

Aylesbury vocational training scheme is one of eight schemes in the Oxford deanery. The current trainers bemoaned the lack of evidence for how they might be 'adding value' to their trainees' learning process. One member of the group (EBP) agreed to make a start by interviewing as many former registrars as possible in order to ascertain their views.

By analysing these semi-structured interviews using a grounded theory methodology, we obtained eight categories of training behaviours, which were arranged with dimensions spanning between 'desired behaviour' and 'less helpful behaviour' (*see* Table 14.1). These categories and dimensions were tested for face validity and content validity by processes that have been described elsewhere.[21]

A more detailed exposition of these categories can be found elsewhere,[22] but if we accept for the moment that they are a valid representation of the perceptions of former learners, then we need to look at how the categories fit with the existing evidence base for training.

Triangulation with other published work

Marinker[14] expanded on the qualities delineated in category 1 (training or education):

> *Training simply prepares the learner to perform tasks already identified and described, by methods which have gained general approval. Training teaches us to solve puzzles, not to solve problems. Education teaches us to solve problems, the nature of which may not be known at the time when the education is taking place, and the solutions to which cannot be seen or even imagined by the teachers.*

Educationalists have begun to tease out some important features of vocational training. Bligh's[23] work suggested that three principal factors influenced GP trainees' readiness to learn:

- enjoyment and enthusiasm for learning
- a positive self-concept as a learner
- a reproducing orientation to learning.

Bligh and Slade[24] went on to conduct interviews at the end of the training year, and they identified six subscales using principal-component analysis. With one exception these appear to fit well with the present research. The

Table 14.1: Categories and dimensions

Category of training behaviour	Desired behaviour	Less helpful behaviour
1 Training or education	*Problem-based approach* Teaching based on approaches to problems which are not limited to present-day contexts	*Emphasis on managing disease* Teaching focused on current policies for disease management
2 Style spectrum	*Wide variety of styles* Learner exposed to different consulting styles and role models in tutorials	*Narrow range of styles* Teaching dominated by personal style and behaviour of trainer
3 Space for reflection	*Encouraging reflective practitioner* Safe environment in which to learn from mistakes	*Protocol-driven behaviour* Black-and-white approach adopted, where learner is expected to adhere to guidelines, and elements of blame culture are likely
4 Modelling personal development and team skills	*Personal development and team management skills taught* Guided learning of skills such as time management, assertiveness and boundary-setting	*No emphasis on team behaviours* Little attempt is made to help learner to understand the importance of teamworking and the areas of personal development that are involved
5 Learning cycles	*Learning cycles completed* A culture exists in the practice where reflection, audit and assessment all promote change and re-evaluation	*Haphazard change* Culture is reactive to external pressures, and there is little evidence of information about the practice inspiring meaningful change
6 Family practice in context	*Contextualised learning* Trainer introduces the broader dimensions of family and health expectations	*Emphasis on presenting problem* Focus remains on sorting and shifting
7 Control and direction	*Learner-centred approach* Trainer encourages progression towards self-directed learning	*Trainer-centred approach* Fails to match style to learner's needs. Rigid structure – fixed diet
8 Feedback	*Sensitive feedback* Both positive and negative feedback is delivered where appropriate, stimulating confidence in the learner, and encouraging change	*Inappropriate criticism* Feedback either inadequate, misplaced or poorly delivered; often not timely or specific enough to be useful to learner

exception occurs where they reported a subscale of trainees' 'desire for clear guidelines', which is at odds with former Aylesbury trainees reporting that they preferred education which encouraged reflection, rather than being driven by protocols or guidelines (see category 1 – training or education).

A Delphi study conducted in South Thames[25] in 1998 on trainers, registrars and non-training principals looked for key attributes of trainers and revealed four factors, namely interpersonal relationships, professional development, personality and teaching quality. It would seem that category 1 (training or education) and category 4 (modelling personal development and team skills) are together of prime importance with regard to these attributes, but it is likely that category 7 (control and direction) and category 8 (feedback) are also highly relevant.

Recent work on the stage theory described in *How Doctors Learn*, by Slotnick,[26] has suggested that there is a preliminary phase of scanning: 'The doctor is aware that problems are "out there". The doctor is alert for problems which he might need to solve and, when potential problems are encountered, he moves on to the next stage.' Slotnick refers to 'Learning Stage 0', where doctors are ready to progress with lifelong learning. Several of the Aylesbury categories would seem to be important in ensuring that general practice registrars are at this stage by the completion of vocational training. These include the following:

- modelling personal development and team skills in the training practice (category 4)
- control and direction (category 7)
- feedback (category 8)
- family practice in context (category 6).

Slotnick concentrates on a stage theory, breaking each stage down to the goals, the discrepancy resolved during that stage, the way in which learning resources are used, the reflection during the stage, and the criteria for successful completion. However, Kolb and Fry[27] viewed learning more in terms of the learning cycle, which was the focus for category 5.

Focus group work at the UKCRA workshop

The contents of this chapter formed the basis of a workshop at the UKCRA conference. Workshop participants were encouraged to come with ideas of behaviours that really add value to registrars' training. Before they were shown any categories from the research work, these experienced educators were asked to contribute their ideas of what might be of lasting value for GP

Table 14.2:   Brainstorming in the UKCRA workshop: what has lasting value?

Brainstorming points on workshop flipchart		Closest matching category from Table 14.1
Mastering evidence-based practice Understanding uncertainty and thriving on it	1	Training or education
Styles as a learning objective	2	Style spectrum
Learning how to know that there is something to reflect on Learning to reflect on things that have gone well	3	Space for reflection

Effective modelling
  Lasting influence of trainer
  From apprenticeship to independence
Recognising one's own limitations
	4	Modelling personal development and team skills

Becoming one's own educational manager Recognising educational needs	5	Learning cycles
Learning about the community of patients	6	Family practice in context
Learner-centred education Learner being valued Managing one's own learning: learning how to learn Being supported	7	Control and direction
High-order teaching skills There were no points on the flipchart which did not match any research category	8	Feeback

registrars. The ideas were recorded on a flipchart, and required negligible 'shoe-horning' on behalf of the presenter to 'fit' the research categories (*see* Table 14.2). (The author recently had a parallel experience when presenting the researched categories to new registrars on the Oxford Deanery Introductory Course. Unprompted, the novice learners also brainstormed compatible points when asked what they thought would be likely to have lasting value from the year ahead.)

Two conclusions may be drawn from this agreement. First, the fact that educators arrive at the same destination having travelled from different ones supports the face validity and construct validity of the research categories. Secondly, it demonstrates that there is nothing startlingly new about the research. Indeed, we might expect the great and the good to be able to suggest appropriate training behaviours, based on their personal observations and experience. Does this mean that the research should be consigned to the dump for reinvented wheels? I suggest not. If education leans forever on intuition rather than evidence, then the task of promoting beneficial changes in training behaviours of the less able educators will indeed be an uphill struggle. However, researched categories that accord well with personal experience are likely to be implementable in the pursuit of improvement.

The presentation of the research categories and dimensions was followed by much interesting discussion. Among the contributions, three stood out as particularly useful.

1   Local differences between district schemes show that teachers can learn to become more effective.
2   Anecdotal evidence suggests that patient-centred doctors are not automatically learner-centred teachers.
3   Hungry GP learners will go in search of educational food. Dependent learners want spoon-feeding (have they missed a window in their development?).

When we think that we know what has lasting value, what do we do about it?

The Aylesbury trainers held a study day to digest the feedback from their former registrars. This was a useful exercise in itself, as the anticipation of possible wounding comments about themselves by former trainees has sensitised trainers when giving feedback to current trainees. There is scope for other trainer groups to obtain meaningful consumer feedback.

Although the categories outlined in Table 4.1 may have a certain face validity and content validity, there should not be any attempt to promote them as helpful training behaviours until there is evidence, beyond the learners' perceptions, to support their usefulness. Work is currently in progress to determine whether these training behaviours could be assessed in training practices. If they are assessable, then a further attempt will be made to relate training behaviours that are deemed to be helpful and those deemed to be less helpful to outcomes in terms of the quality of the trainees' later performance in practice. This has to be the gold standard for determining where training is adding value.

Conclusion

It seems that there is indeed a piece missing from the jigsaw of general practice. It is not just a piece of sky, which could almost be ignored, but rather it is a piece of critical focal interest – the bit that general practice trainers everywhere are keen to look at. *What are we doing that adds value to our registrars' learning?* The genuine (evidence-based) piece is missing, and to date in putting the jigsaw together we have had to rely on temporary or makeshift substitute pieces (the notions of the good and the great, and the unproven ideas of committed educators) to hold the jigsaw in place. We are at last able to determine the shape of the missing piece, and work is now in progress to construct a full-colour replica. What will it look like?

References

1 Anyon P (1987) *An Evaluation of the New Zealand Family Medicine Training Programme*. Royal New Zealand College of General Practitioners, Wellington.

2 Freer CB and Reid ME (1978) A survey of past trainees (vocational training forum). *Update*. **16**: 1461–8.

3 Martys CR (1979) Some trainees' views on vocational training. *Update*. **18**: 1079–81.

4 Duncan P (1994) Evaluation of the GPVTP. *N Z Fam Physician*. **21**: 186–8.

5 Crawley HS and Levin JB (1990) Training for general practice: result of a survey into the general practitioner trainee scheme. *BMJ*. **300**: 911–15.

6 Short NL (1987) Vocational training for general practice in Dartford 1971–1982: an assessment. *Med Teacher*. **9**: 193–9.

7 Ronalds C, Douglas A and Gray DP *et al.* (1981) Fourth National Trainee Conference, Exeter, 1980. *Reports, Recommendations and Questionnaire. Occasional Paper 18*. Royal College of General Practitioners, London.

8 Hilton S (1981) Looking back on a trainee year. *Practitioner*. **225**: 443–4.

9 Whitfield MJ (1966) Training for general practice: result of a survey into the general practitioner trainee scheme. *BMJ*. **1**: 663–7.

10 Thornham JR (1980) A survey of ex-trainees. *J R Coll Gen Pract*. **30**: 725–8.

11 Freeman F and Byrne PS (1976) *The Assessment of Vocational Training for General Practice. Reports from General Practice*. Royal College of General Practitioners, London.

12 Kelly DR and Murray T (1991) Twenty years of vocational training in the West of Scotland: the practice component. *Br J Gen Pract*. **41**: 492–5.

13 Bain J (1996) Vocational training: the end or the beginning? *Br J Gen Pract*. **46**: 328–30.

14 Marinker M (1992) Assessment of postgraduate medical education – future directions. In: M Lawrence and P Pritchard (eds) *General Practitioner Education: UK and Nordic Perspectives*. Springer Verlag, London, 75–80.

15 Royal College of General Practitioners (1985) *What Sort of Doctor? Assessing Quality of Care in General Practice*. Royal College of General Practitioners, London.

16 Calman K (1994) The profession of medicine. *BMJ*. **309**: 1140–3.

17 Southgate L (1994) Freedom and discipline: clinical practice and the assessment of clinical competence. *Br J Gen Pract.* **44**: 87–92.

18 Van Leeuwen YD, Mol S and Pollemans MC *et al.* (1995) Change in knowledge of general practice during their professional career. *Fam Pract.* **12**: 313–17.

19 Smith F, Singleton A and Hilton S (1998) General practitioners' continuing education: a review of policies, strategies and effectiveness, and their implications for the future. *Br J Gen Pract.* **48**: 1689–95.

20 Hindmarsh JH, Coster GD and Gilbert C (1998) Are vocationally trained general practitioners better GPs? A review of research designs and outcomes. *Med Educ.* **32**: 244–54.

21 Strauss A and Corbin J (1998) *Basics of Qualitative Research Techniques and Procedures for Developing Grounded Theory.* Sage, Thousand Oaks, CA.

22 Peile E, Easton G and Johnson N (2000) The year in a training practice: what has lasting value? *Med Teacher.* In press.

23 Bligh GH (1992) Independent learning among general practice trainees: an initial survey. *Med Educ.* **26**: 497–502.

24 Bligh J and Slade P (1996) A questionnaire examining learning in general practice. *Med Educ.* **30**: 65–70.

25 Munro N, Hornung R and McAleer S (1998) What are the key attributes of a good general practice trainer? *Educ Gen Pract.* **9**: 263–70.

26 Slotnick H (1999) How doctors learn: physicians' self-directed learning episodes. *Acad Med.* **74**: 1106–17.

27 Kolb D and Fry R (1975) Towards an applied theory of experiential learning. In: C Cooper (ed.) *Theories of Group Processes.* John Wiley & Sons, Chichester.

15

Problem-based learning: a valuable educational tool for use in the primary healthcare team and in training in general practice

Paul Downey and Dec O'Brien

Problem-based learning (PBL) is not new. It has been used extensively in Canada and the USA for many years,[1] and more recently it has been used in undergraduate medical education in the UK.[2]

Following some experience of PBL in the USA and Australia, we have been using PBL on the Hereford vocational training scheme for the last three years.[3] Encouraged by its success and efficacy, we have produced a PBL facilitator's pack for the Hereford vocational training scheme, which has now been used by many course organisers both in the West Midlands region and further afield.

As we are full-time general practitioners, it seemed only natural to try PBL in our own practices. Again it proved to be a great success. We have now produced a PBL facilitator's pack for the primary healthcare team (PHCT).

What is PBL?

- PBL uses cases or 'problems' to identify the learning needs of an individual or a group. The individual or group then addresses these learning needs.
- PBL is not problem-solving, although this might be part of the process.
- PBL is not significant event analysis, although there are some similarities.

What do you need?

PBL has three requirements:

- a problem
- a facilitator
- an individual or a group.

The problem is essentially the 'trigger' material that is designed to provoke discussion in the group. Considerable skill is required in problem design. Cases can contain a mixture of clinical, ethical and management issues.

The facilitator is an important figure who must have both a good understanding of PBL and the skills required to run a small group. The facilitator's job is essentially to keep the group focused on identifying learning issues – not providing solutions to the case or letting group members demonstrate how clever or powerful they are.

The group should ideally consist of six to ten people. Obviously in the PHCT the group should be multidisciplinary.

What happens?

The group selects a case and sits down to discuss it. Ideally they should have 1.5–2 hours of protected time. The facilitator reminds the group of the task (i.e. to use the case to identify learning issues). A reader is nominated, and a volunteer is also needed who briefly records the proceedings. We use the following three headings.

FACTS   IDEAS   LEARNING ISSUES

Both the record-keeper and the reader take part in the discussion.

At the UKCRA conference a small group of eminent medical educators role-played a PHCT and discussed a couple of pages of a sample case (*see* Boxes 15.1 and 15.2). We could probably have spent two hours on page 1!

As the discussion continues, learning issues are identified and recorded. The learning issues will be relevant to and owned by the individual or group. The group discusses, reflects and thus learns together about issues which are important to them. This is PBL, but we are only halfway through the process.

Education is pointless unless it results in change. Having identified the learning issues, the group then decides which ones they are going to address and how they are going to do this.

Our UKCRA group might have decided to look at procedures for handling violent patients, to update on the management of ectopic pregnancy, to

---

Box 15.1:   Page 1 of sample case

10.30 Saturday morning, emergency surgery.
Dr Bernard Banks is on. Sally Payne is the duty receptionist.
Sally is 'stressed' because Dr Banks is in his usual bad mood. He hates doing
Saturday mornings.
It is busy.
Jimmy Cousins approaches the reception desk.
'I've come for my methadone scrip. I couldn't make it yesterday, I was ill.'

Learning issues for our group:
*   *opening hours and service provision*
*   *is methadone prescribing appropriate for primary care?*
*   *violent patients*
*   *health and safety issues with regard to working solo*
*   *stereotyping patients*
*   *stress and its management*
*   *sick doctors*
*   *communication issues in practice*
*   *practice protocols.*

Box 15.2:   Page 2 of sample case

10.30 Saturday morning. Dr Banks is in surgery.
Amy Layton, aged 18 years, works at the local chicken factory. She lives in a
bed-sit.
Amy has lower abdominal pain. She has had it for four days but it is worse
today. She is otherwise well.
She always has a slight discharge.
She has regular sexual intercourse and occasionally uses condoms.
She thinks her last period was about three weeks ago.
She had a termination when she was 15 years old.
Her parents divorced when she was six years old.

Learning issues for our group
*   *receptionist triage*
*   *training receptionists*
*   *diagnosis of ectopic pregnancy*
*   *medical emergencies*
*   *use of chaperones*
*   *medicalisation of problems*
*   *access to investigations*
*   *access to secondary care.*

undertake an audit of non-attenders, to review the literature on the efficacy of methadone prescribing, or to reflect on ways of dealing with a potentially 'burnt-out' or depressed partner.

Having allocated specific learning issues, the group then decides on a deadline for reporting back. This follow-up session might take place two weeks later. Individuals report back to the group and changes will be suggested. It is not unusual for the follow-up session to give rise to further learning issues.

The process can be summarised by the flow-chart shown in Figure 15.1.

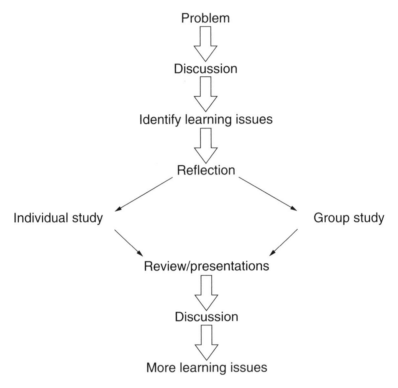

Figure 15.1:   Hereford PBL model.

The Hereford experience

We have used PBL extensively on our VTS. The half-day release course is frequently labelled as a 'cosy talking-shop'. However, PBL has ensured that ours certainly is not.

PBL has many benefits, which include the following.

- The course is based on the needs of the learners.
- It encourages true adult learning (i.e. learning issues are truly owned and addressed by group members).

- It encourages reflection.
- Huge areas of traditional curriculum are covered effectively.
- Teamwork is enhanced.
- Group skills are learned.
- Presentation skills are developed.
- It is hard work but great fun!

Thanks to support and encouragement from our PCG, PBL is being used widely in PHCTs in Herefordshire. If anything, our experience of using PBL in the PHCT is even more exciting. In some cases, PHCTs are sitting down and learning together for the first time. Learning issues which are relevant to that team are being identified and addressed. Clinical governance issues are covered, as are some issues identified in our local health improvement programme strategy. Team members who may not previously have had a voice are being listened to. In particular, non-medical members of the team are taking on learning issues and suggesting and making changes. Some individuals feel 'important and valued' for the first time in their careers. Interestingly, we have found that it is the doctors who are often the slowest to get involved!

Conclusion

Problem-based learning is a well-established educational tool. It is inexpensive, effective and fun. It lends itself readily to use both on the VTS and in the PHCT. It can be a powerful force for promoting change in a practice and thus for improving patient care.

The facilitator's packs

We have produced two facilitator's packs, one designed specifically for the VTS and the other for the PHCT.

The Hereford PBL pack for PHCTs is an 120-page A4-bound folder containing a history of the development of PBL. It also contains a 'how to do it guide' and an introduction to facilitating a small group, as well as eight cases. Each case unravels over about 10 pages, and provides four hours of educational activity. The cases are designed to be of relevance to all members of the PHCT, and they cover clinical, administrative and ethical issues.

In Hereford the pack has been PGEA-approved for doctors.

These packs are also available in CD-ROM format.

For more information on the facilitator's packs please contact:
Mrs Ann Lane
John Ross Postgraduate Medical Centre
County Hospital
Hereford HR1 2ER
Tel 01432 364025
Fax 01432 355265
Email hfd.pgmc@dial.pipex.com

or visit our website
www.problembasedlearning.co.uk

References

1   Lowry S (1993) *Medical Education.* BMJ Publishing, London.

2   Robinson LA, Spencer JA and Jones RH (1994) Contribution of undergraduate departments of general practice to teaching and their plans for curriculum development *Br J Gen Pract.* **44**: 489–91.

3   Downey P and O'Brien D (1999) Problem-based learning in GP vocational training. *Educ Gen Pract.* **10**: 265–71.

16

Using a chronological format for feedback

Lesley Millard

Introduction

This paper reports on a workshop which had two main objectives, namely to provide opportunities to compare a chronological format for giving feedback with a 'what went well/less well' structure, and to identify specific features associated with chronological feedback.

Outline of the session

Participants were asked to introduce themselves, outline their interest in the workshop, and state what experiences they had had of a 'what went well/ what went less well' approach and other structures for giving feedback.

The meaning of 'chronological feedback' was outlined. The term refers to comments which are made in the same time sequence as the behaviour, which is observed (once the learner has made his or her comments), and the person giving feedback reports on what could be seen to be happening at the time. The intention is, as far as possible, to hold up a mirror which reflects what occurred, leaving the learner to make judgements, and separating suggestions and advice from the feedback process.

The important educational attributes of chronological feedback are as follows.

- It makes the perceptions and feelings of the learner the starting point.
- It encourages observational comments.
- It helps learners to rerun what was in their mind at the time.
- It acknowledges the complexity of interactions.
- It promotes dialogue which leads to the learner's own judgements and action planning.

During the workshop, the following examples of observational and more judgemental feedback were offered to the participants.

- *I noticed you were looking down at your papers as she began to speak.*
- I didn't think you were really listening to him.
- *You did not ask any questions for the first few minutes or so.*
- You put the patient at his ease.
- *You spoke twice while she was speaking about the pain.*
- Things didn't seem to go so well after you had examined him.
- *You smiled a lot towards the end.*

Note that the more direct, observational comments appear in italic, and the sentences are independent of each other.

After the introduction, a short role-play of a GP tutor helping a general practitioner to explore his continuing professional development needs was used to provide an opportunity for the group members to practise making observations in a time sequence, while at the same time seeking to suspend judgements as far as possible. Comments arising from the exercise indicated that it was not difficult to decide whether a particular behaviour was helpful or unhelpful, but instead simply to note what was seen and to feed this back to the learner, so that he or she could explain what was intended.

The participants discussed the way in which observational feedback, given in the time sequence in which the behaviour occurred, can open up dialogue with a learner. This approach was felt to be less likely to generate defensiveness than a 'what went well/what went less well' format. The example of inter-ruptions was given. If a GP registrar interrupts a patient, the trainer might view this as undesirable. However, if the feedback he or she gives is merely to say 'I noticed you spoke over the patient', then this leaves the GP registrar free to explain 'Yes, I did that deliberately as I thought it was very important that I really understood what he was saying then', or to say 'Did I? Oh dear, I hadn't realised'. Either explanation is possible, but only the registrar knows what was the intention behind the behaviour. Once the intention has been explained, the trainer is in a better position to help the registrar than if he or she labels the behaviour as helpful or unhelpful and conveys this judgement in the way he or she gives the feedback.

A more observational approach (although of course some degree of judge-ment is inevitably present) is supported by using a chronological format for offering feedback – this happened, followed by this and then that. The reported behaviours are not pre-labelled as helpful or unhelpful, and the learner can be helped to replay what happened in their mind's eye and thus get back in touch with their original feelings and intentions, even when a video recording may not be available.

Summary

A chronological structure for feedback supports observational (i.e. less judgemental) feedback and offers a more learner-centred approach than more judgemental formats. It recognises and honours the complexity of human interactions. Further discussion on chronological feedback appears in Millard L (2000) Teaching the teachers: ways of improving teaching and identifying areas for development. *Annals Rheum Dis.* **59**(10): 760–4.

17

Audit and summative assessment: completing the cycle

Murray Lough

Summative assessment of general practice registrars has been a professionally led system in the UK since September 1996, and it acquired legal status in January 1998. The submission of an audit project is one of the four components of the assessment process.

The current marking schedule uses five criteria to assess an audit, which does not require a completed cycle to demonstrate minimum competence in the understanding of basic audit method.

The current assessment system is a screening process where pass/refer decisions are based on professional judgements guided by the five criteria. Combining assessor judgements and using a cascade referral system to a second level of more experienced assessors for doubtful projects maximises the likelihood of detecting a poor project (sensitivity) while trading off a number of borderline projects which enter the referral system and will ultimately pass (specificity). A project reviewed at second level, if it is still not demonstrating minimum competence of an understanding of basic audit method, will be sent back to the registrar for resubmission. All projects which fail after resubmission are further reviewed by a national panel of second-level assessors from other regions which acts as a quality control for the whole process.

Development of this system for assessing a completed audit cycle

In June 1997, 144 trainers in the West of Scotland were asked to prioritise the 14 elements that had previously been agreed upon in the constitution of a registrar's audit project.

Ten complete audit cycles and ten incomplete audit cycles were chosen at random from the 1998 audit projects submitted for summative assessment in the previous year, and were marked by 26 experienced assessors. The ability of single, double and treble marking to identify a completed audit cycle was assessed.

All 57 registrars who began their training in August 1997 underwent a pilot exercise of the completed audit cycle, using eight criteria with two assessors independently marking their projects. A subsequent check of the sensitivity and specificity of the instrument was made using 11 projects – nine (out of 42) passed at first level and two (out of seven) referred by second level for resubmission. All assessors and registrars were asked for their opinions about their perceived difficulty with the new system.

Discussion

The move to a completed audit cycle was regarded as a positive exercise by trainers, registrars and assessors. Trainers were more positive about teaching a completed audit cycle, registrars had already been completing audit cycles in significant numbers, and assessors found the new marking schedule with eight criteria easier to use.

One problem with the previous marking schedule was the criterion 'detailed proposals for change', the results of which were often quite difficult to assess. These difficulties were overcome by completing the cycle. Involving two rather than three markers at first level, while retaining the sensitivity of the instrument, reduced the workload and resulted in smaller, more focused projects.

In total, 265 audit projects have been submitted in the West of Scotland over the past three years, with just over 70% passing at first level and around 10% requiring resubmission. Of two data collections, 47% are completed in less than three months, with 92% being completed in less than five months. The number of registrars assessing four or more criteria fell from 33% prior to the completion of a cycle to 14% when a completed audit cycle was needed. Furthermore, one-third of registrars assessed one criterion prior to a completed cycle, with nearly 50% assessing this on the completion of a cycle.

Trainers are now much more confident about the teaching of audit, and this is reflected in the quality of the projects now being seen. However, an adequate trainer support network is vital for those who may be less experienced and therefore less confident, and it should be emphasised that the trainer may not be the most appropriate person in the practice to teach the subject. Given the tight timescale and the pressure of many other educational activities in the training year, the concept of an audit calendar should be encouraged to allow systematic checks on a registrar's progress with their audit throughout their time in the practice.

Future issues

Standards in the teaching and execution of an audit project are rising. In order to ensure that an audit project still provides adequate discrimination in the summative assessment process, and due to the need to avoid a trend towards minimisation, further issues of audit method may need to be addressed. In the West of Scotland the following three areas are under consideration:

- stopping a resubmission
- sample size technique
- confidence intervals.

With revalidation requiring a knowledge of basic audit method, and a tightening of the Joint Committee criterion for audit in training practices, the move to a completed audit cycle has been very timely. There are implications in the lessons that have been learned from this journey both for vocationally training SHOs and, perhaps more urgently, for non-training practices.

This raises the question of whether all principals in general practice should be required to demonstrate satisfactorily a completed audit cycle and a significant event analysis.

18

The National Project Marking Schedule: an alternative to audit for the written submission component of summative assessment

Jamie Bahrami, Philip Nolan and Alison Evans

The National Project Marking Schedule (NPMS) has been approved by the JCPTGP as an alternative to audit for the written submission component of summative assessment, and is available from 1 April 2000. Registrars are now able to submit a wider range of projects than previously, including audit.

A project is defined as a self-directed piece of learning which:

- addresses a defined problem
- is related to previous work
- presents qualitative or quantitative findings
- interprets these findings
- draws conclusions from the evidence presented.

The core competencies to be tested will be those originally defined by the JCPTGP for the written submission, namely:

- the ability to construct a logical argument and communicate it in written English
- the ability to plan and sustain activity over time.

How is the National Project Marking Schedule different?

Registrars may submit a wider range of work, including the following:

- a small research study (e.g. questionnaire, notes review or interview study)
- an audit of any type
- a literature review
- a case study
- a proposal for a new service in the practice
- a discussion paper.

Registrars are therefore encouraged to be creative, and are not constrained by the step-by-step approach of the old marking schedule. The NPMS describes each level of achievement, so that registrars have a clear idea of what is required and are encouraged to aim higher than a level of minimum competence. If a registrar has to resubmit, he or she can see which areas need attention. The criteria on the NPMS are marked on a scale rather than on an 'all or nothing basis', which allows markers to give credit for what is presented. The pass mark is 18 or more out of a possible 30 marks, with a score of not less than two on any criterion. A further difference is that the project must contain appropriate references to the literature in order to pass.

Validity and reliability

The schedule was developed by general practice educators with experience of assessing projects, and it was then sent out to a national sample of trainers and course organisers, as well as Directors of Postgraduate General Practice Education and associate advisers, for their feedback and comments. The majority of the 186 educators who replied agreed with the criteria used and the description of the level of minimum competence.[1] Several helpful suggestions were received, and the schedule was modified in the light of these. The 17 markers in the Yorkshire deanery, who each marked 20 projects, carried out reliability testing. There was good agreement between markers, with high sensitivity and specificity.[2]

The marking system

The system of marking is the same as that for the other summative assessment instrument for marking audit projects. The project is marked by three 'first'-level markers, and is sent to two 'second'-level markers if it is referred by any of the 'first'-level markers. The two 'second'-level markers must agree the score on each criterion, and therefore on pass or 'refer'. If the project is referred, it is returned to the registrar with a copy of the marking schedule and an invitation to resubmit. The same 'second'-level markers mark resubmitted projects. Projects that are referred after resubmission are submitted to national markers who make the final decision with regard to pass or fail. If the project fails, the comments of all of the markers are sent to the registrar's new trainer if additional training is undertaken.

Implementing the National Project Marking Schedule

An information pack for registrars is available on request from the Yorkshire deanery. This includes instructions on how to submit the work, as well as guidance on how to produce a project for the National Project Marking Schedule. The content of this pack is included in the information pack for general practice educators, which is also available from the Yorkshire deanery. In addition, the pack for educators contains the instructions for markers.

Deaneries that only have a small number of registrars who wish to submit a project may send the submissions to the Yorkshire deanery for marking. Yorkshire markers will then claim their fees directly from the registrar's deanery. Deaneries that wish to train their own markers should follow the steps suggested in the pack *Advice to Deaneries*, which gives advice on the training of markers, and also includes projects which can be used for training and calibration. All markers should attend two calibration meetings each year, which should be arranged in their own deanery. Second-level markers must also attend one national calibration meeting each year. Meetings will be held in Edinburgh, Leeds and London in autumn each year.

Quality control

The same system of quality control will be used as for the other schedule. A random selection of 10% of submitted projects should be sent to the national markers for remarking. All markers should receive feedback on their performance compared with their colleagues on a quarterly basis. They should also receive the results of the quality control exercise. Markers who usually appear to be inconsistent in their performance should be offered further training and demonstrate consistency in calibration exercises before they mark any further projects for assessment purposes.

Conclusion

Since the introduction of summative assessment, we have seen little if any original project work undertaken by registrars. We hope that the introduction of the National Project Marking Schedule will rekindle the creative spirit, and as our experience of more different types of projects grows we will be able to offer an even wider range of written submission.

References

1   Evans A, Singleton S, Nolan P and Hall W (1996) Summative assessment of general practice registrars' projects: deciding on criteria and developing a marking schedule. *Educ Gen Pract.* **7**: 229–36.

2   Evans A, Nolan P, Bogle S, Hall W and Bahrami J (1997) Summative assessment of general practice registrars' projects: reliability of the Yorkshire schedule. *Educ Gen Pract.* **8**: 40–7.

19

The videotape assessment of consulting skills for summative assessment: the single route through MRCGP and summative assessment

Steve Field

Introduction

Since summative assessment began in 1996, registrars, trainers, course organisers and Directors of Postgraduate General Practice Education have frequently complained about the waste of time that occurs during the training year as a result of preparing for two different systems of assessing videotapes of consultations. At last a solution has been found that seems to satisfy everybody. The result should be that registrars will be able to concentrate on the 'gold standard' of the MRCGP examination and have more time to devote to their other learning needs during their training year.

In the summer of 2000, the JCPTGP approved a pass in the MRCGP video assessment of consultations as acceptable for summative assessment purposes. Registrars are now therefore able to prepare a single tape which, once submitted to their deanery office, will be passed through the RCGP's assessment process. If the video fails the MRCGP assessment, it will be submitted anonymously to the deanery's summative assessment process. Registrars will continue to have the choice of sending their tape through the deanery's summative assessment process or sitting the Yorkshire/Leicester simulated patient test. Although there is still consternation in some quarters that the MRCGP examination's method is not the only test of consulting skills allowed for summative assessment purposes, overall the agreement on the single route should make the whole process much simpler for the vast majority of GP registrars.

The single route (see Figure 19.1)

This has been made as straightforward as possible. The registrars simply have to prepare a single videotape for both systems and complete an MRCGP workbook, consent forms and a summative assessment video declaration form (countersigned by their trainer). Those who wish to have their tape assessed for the MRCGP examination must also apply to the RCGP in advance and pay the fee. The deanery offices will handle all videotapes that are submitted for summative assessment purposes. This includes tapes that registrars also wish to use for the single route to MRCGP and summative assessment. The deanery office will pass the tapes on to the RCGP if the registrar has indicated that that is what they wish to happen (see Box 19.1).

About 25–30% of tapes assessed by the RCGP will fail. These will be sent back to the deaneries and put into the first-level summative assessment pathway. Tapes that have gone via this route will be indistinguishable from tapes sent by registrars who have elected not to sit the MRCGP examination.

The deanery offices will issue all summative assessment results, and MRCGP results will be released by the RCGP separately. Registrars' rights to appeal, resubmit tapes and extend training will remain unchanged.

By managing the tapes in the deanery offices it is hoped that the summative assessment process will not be adversely affected by the opportunity afforded to registrars to have their tape assessed by the RCGP. The GP registrar will continue to pay for the MRCGP examination, and summative assessment will continue to be funded by the deaneries.

Box 19.1:   The single route – what needs to be submitted?

- A letter from the registrar stating their intention to take the single route for MRCGP and summative assessment
- One videotape of the registrar's own consultations
- Copies of consent forms for each consultation
- One MRCGP workbook (2001 edition or later)
- A completed summative assessment video declaration form

Registrars should aim for the 'gold standard' – the MRCGP examination

The MRCGP performance criteria may look complicated, but they have been developed as part of an educational tool to help doctors to look more closely at their consultations, and to help them to improve their consulting skills. The

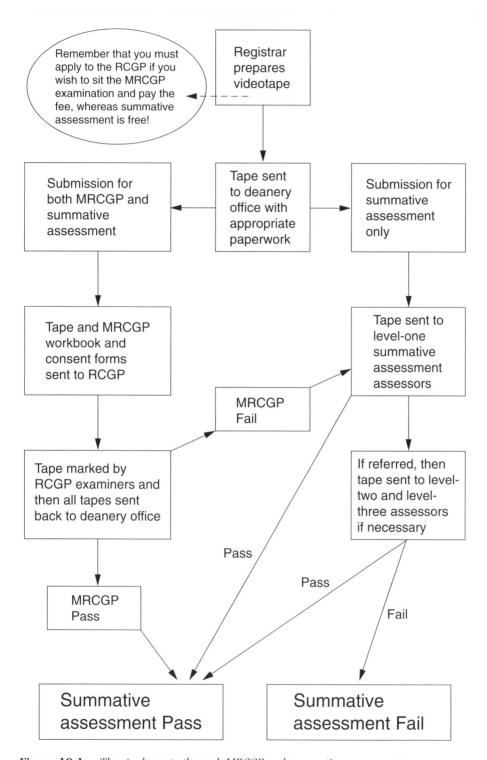

Figure 19.1:   The single route through MRCGP and summative assessment.

MRCGP examiners do not want to encourage particular styles of behaviour but rather to encourage effective task-based consulting. By routinely using the performance criteria as a tool to assess their own consultations, registrars will not only start to improve their effectiveness as general practitioners, but will also be preparing themselves for their video submission.

The development of the MRCGP assessment method

The RCGP believes that competence in consulting has three basic attributes.

1 Competence can be pre-defined.
2 Competence is about outcomes, not behaviours.
3 Competence is either present or absent.

Basically the assessment looks at whether or not the registrar demonstrates competence in their consultations.

The MRCGP assessment method was devised by general practitioners under the guidance of Dr Peter Tate, who was part of Pendleton's[1] team, whose task-oriented approach to the consultation forms the bedrock of most registrars' training on consulting skills. The world literature was searched and a consensus was reached on what competences were demonstrated in effective consultations. These were called *units* (*see* Box 19.2). Each of these units was subdivided into elements. For example, in unit one, *discover the reasons for the patient's attendance*, there were four elements (*see* Box 19.3).

Box 19.2:   Units of the consultation used in the MRCGP examination

1 Discover the reasons for the patient's attendance.
2 Define the clinical problem(s).
3 Explain the problem(s) to the patient.
4 Address the patient's problem(s).
5 Make effective use of the consultation.

Box 19.3:   Elements of the consultation used in the MRCGP examination

1 Elicit the patient's account of the symptom(s) that caused him or her to consult the doctor.
2 Obtain relevant items of social and occupational circumstances.
3 Explore the patient's health understanding.
4 Enquire about continuing problems.

It was felt that the elements were too broad to be assessed reliably even at this level. An even more specific level was defined, called the *Performance criteria* (PC). Each element has one or more performance criteria. Members of the video development group of the MRCGP panel of examiners (who were practising general practitioners) derived the PCs. Thus for the unit *discover the reasons for the patient's attendance* and the element *elicit the patient's account of the symptoms which caused him or her to consult the doctor*, there are two performance criteria.

1   The doctor encourages the patient's contribution at appropriate points in the consultation.
2   The doctor responds to cues.

The full definition in addition to the five units has 16 elements and 21 performance criteria (*see* Figure 19.2).

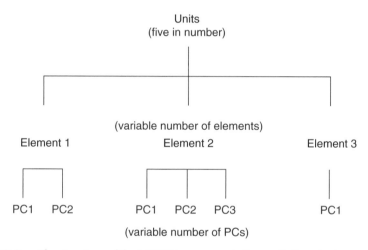

Figure 19.2:   The structure of the MRCGP assessment of consultations instrument.[4]

Following a pilot exercise, the entire panel of examiners was consulted to define the PCs that would need to be demonstrated in order to achieve a 'pass' or a 'pass with merit'. These were incorporated into the examination in May 1998.

The MRCGP assessment process

The examiners watch the first five consultations, and the final two will only be reviewed if sufficient evidence of competence in the first five has been demonstrated. The candidate fails if there is insufficient evidence demonstrated in the seven consultations, or if the tape demonstrates evidence of major clinical errors. Pass with merit is achieved if sufficient evidence of the performance criteria preceded by (M) is found in the first five consultations. For those registrars who have chosen the single route, summative assessment assessors in the registrar's deanery would then mark a failed MRCGP tape (*see* Box 19.4).

Box 19.4: The MRCGP examination assessment of consulting skills module: the units, elements and performance criteria

UNIT 1 **Discover the reasons for a patient's attendance**

Element A. ELICIT THE PATIENT'S ACCOUNT OF THE SYMPTOM(S) WHICH MADE HIM OR HER TURN TO THE DOCTOR

(P) PC: *The doctor encourages the patient's contribution at appropriate points in the consultation*

(P) PC: *The doctor responds to cues*

Element B. OBTAIN RELEVANT ITEMS OF SOCIAL AND OCCUPATIONAL CIRCUMSTANCES

(P) PC: *The doctor elicits appropriate details to place the complaint(s) in a social and psychological context*

Element C. EXPLORE THE PATIENT'S HEALTH UNDERSTANDING

(M) PC: *The doctor takes the patient's health understanding into account*

Element D. ENQUIRE ABOUT CONTINUING PROBLEMS

PC: *The doctor obtains enough information to assess whether a continuing complaint represents an issue, which must be addressed in this consultation*

UNIT 2 **Define the clinical problem(s)**

Element A. OBTAIN ADDITIONAL INFORMATION ABOUT SYMPTOMS AND DETAILS OF MEDICAL HISTORY

(P) PC: *The doctor obtains sufficient information for no serious condition to be missed*

PC: *The doctor shows evidence of generating and testing hypotheses*

Element B. ASSESS THE CONDITION OF THE PATIENT BY APPROPRIATE PHYSICAL OR MENTAL EXAMINATION

(P) PC: *The doctor chooses an examination which is likely to confirm or disprove hypotheses which could reasonably have been formed OR to address a patient's concern*

Element C. MAKE A WORKING DIAGNOSIS

(P) PC: *The doctor appears to make a clinically appropriate working diagnosis*

UNIT 3 **Explain the problem(s) to the patient**

Element A. SHARE THE FINDINGS WITH THE PATIENT

(P) PC: *The doctor explains the diagnosis, management and effects of treatment*

Element B. TAILOR THE EXPLANATION TO THE PATIENT
(P) PC: *The doctor explains in language appropriate to the patient*
(M) PC: *The doctor's explanation takes account of some or all of the patient's elicited beliefs*
Element C. ENSURE THAT THE EXPLANATION IS UNDERSTOOD AND ACCEPTED BY THE PATIENT
(M) PC: *The doctor seeks to confirm the patient's understanding*

UNIT 4 **Address the patient's problem(s)**
Element A. ASSESS THE SEVERITY OF THE PRESENTING PROBLEM(S)
PC: *The doctor differentiates between problems of differing degrees of severity and manages each appropriately*
Element B. CHOOSE AN APPROPRIATE FORM OF MANAGEMENT
(P) PC: *The doctor's management plan is appropriate for the working diagnosis, reflecting a good understanding of modern accepted medical practice*
Element C. INVOLVE THE PATIENT IN THE MANAGEMENT PLAN TO THE APPROPRIATE EXTENT
(P) PC: *The doctor shares management options with the patient*

UNIT 5 **Make effective use of the consultation**
Element A. MAKE EFFICIENT USE OF RESOURCES
PC: *The doctor makes sensible use of available time, and suggests further consultation as appropriate*
PC: *The doctor makes appropriate use of other health professionals through investigations, referrals, etc.*
(P) PC: *The doctor's prescribing behaviour is appropriate*
Element B. ESTABLISH A RELATIONSHIP WITH THE PATIENT
(P) PC: *The patient and doctor appear to have established a rapport*
Element C. GIVE OPPORTUNISTIC HEALTH PROMOTION ADVICE
PC: *The doctor deals appropriately with at-risk factors within the consultation*

The summative assessment process

All tapes that ultimately fail summative assessment will have gone through the full summative assessment procedures. Those registrars who have asked to be assessed by the RCGP will have their tapes assessed for summative assessment purposes if they fail at MRCGP level. About 25–30% doctors fail at MRCGP level, and 4–6% fail summative assessment annually.

The summative assessment process is much simpler than the RCGP's assessment procedure and is set at a lower level of minimal competence. Although the assessors use a marking schedule to help them to make a judgement, there is no numerical scoring system (*see* Box 19.5). The assessments are made at three levels. At the first level, two assessors within the deanery view the tape independently. If they are happy with it they can pass it, but they are encouraged to refer on to the second-level assessors if they have any doubts about its acceptability. If either or both assessors refer the tape, two second-level assessors review it, again within the deanery. They can either pass the tape or refer it on to two third-level assessors who are randomly drawn from a national pool. They review the tape together with the written comments of the first- and second-level assessors. If they feel that the registrar is acceptable they pass the tape. If not, they fail the registrar and then the Director of Postgraduate GP Education will become involved in advising the registrar that they require a period of extra training.

Box 19.5: The UKCRA summative assessment criteria

Listening: The GP registrar should identify and elucidate the reason or reasons for the patient's attendance. Credible and mutually acceptable plans should be negotiated with the patient.

Action: The GP registrar should take appropriate action to identify the patient's problem or problems. Investigations and referral should be reasonable. Help should be sought where necessary. The patient's problem should be managed appropriately.

Understanding: The GP registrar should demonstrate in the logbook that he or she understands the process and outcome of the consultation. Individual action should be explained. Obvious shortcomings in the consultations should be identified, and relevant background should be mentioned.

Error: If a major error is noted in patient management, or if a series of minor errors is noted, the GP registrar may be referred. (A major error is one which causes actual or potential harm to the patient; a minor error only causes inconvenience.)

Tips on how to prepare

Start early

It is important that the registrars discuss the UKCRA summative assessment and the MRCGP procedures with their trainer at the beginning of the training year. The trainer's role is to ensure that the registrar is given the best chance of passing. The trainer also has access to the local course organisers and

Associate Directors who provide additional support if there are difficulties. In addition, local MRCGP examiners are a valuable resource.

Summative assessment procedures are only tests of minimal competence, and registrars should aim at the higher standard of the MRCGP examination. There should be no difficulty in passing either assessment if the registrar works hard, discusses their learning needs with their trainer and course organiser, and does not panic. The key is to prepare well and start early in the registrar year.

It is important to start taping as many consultations as possible early in the training year. Many registrars organise surgeries that help receptionists get into a routine. Receptionists have an essential role in supporting patients in all of this, and in reducing the number of patients who refuse to give consent. Lengthening your appointment times is also helpful.

Background reading

There is no shortage of information on summative assessment and the MRCGP examination. *Training Update* is a valuable source of up-to-date information, and the *Practitioner* also regularly includes information on the MRCGP examination. Deaneries provide details of what is required for summative assessment, and when the registrar applies to sit the MRCGP's assessment module, they receive the comprehensive workbook and examination regulations. The training packages *Watching You, Watching Me... Consulting Skills and Summative Assessment in General Practice* (second edition)[2] and *Those Things You Say... Consulting Skills and the MRCGP Examination*[3] are excellent. They include comprehensive workbooks and a videotape that analyse the individual performance criteria and provide examples of excellent consulting practice. Peter Tate's *The Doctor's Communication Handbook*,[4] is a valuable aid to learning about communication skills, and Roger Neighbour's seminal text *The Inner Consultation*[5] is an important resource that will help the registrar to prepare for their assessment.

Technical aspects

The registrar should aim to produce a tape with the highest technical quality possible. Although videotapes of extremely poor quality are rejected, in other cases poor sound and vision make it difficult for the examiners to make an assessment. It is easier to see and hear your demonstrated competences if the sound and vision are good – and it is therefore easier to pass! The commonest fault found on candidates' videotapes is poor sound, usually because the microphone is on the camera. This means that all sounds in the room (and outside) are amplified, making the voices of the doctor and patient part of a larger cacophony of sound. A desktop microphone solves this problem. The printer also sounds like a machine-gun on some tapes, and it can obscure an important part of the consultation. The doctor and patient should both be in view, as this helps to highlight non-verbal cues which can be missed if you cannot see the faces of the participants. Backlighting is also a potential problem – beware the window behind the doctor or patient (*see* Box 19.6).

Box 19.6:   The videotape

- The registrar should produce a tape of their own consultations on a standard VHS videotape (it is advisable for registrars to keep a copy of their videotape).
- A clock or time stamp should be clearly visible on the videotape.
- The tape should be of sufficient length to satisfy summative assessment needs – two hours of consultations are required.
- The first seven consultations will be marked by the MRCGP examiners.
- Only consultations for which patients have given their consent should be submitted.
- Consultations should exhibit a sufficient level of challenge to allow a decision to be made about competence.

Ethical issues

Doctors should behave ethically at all times, and being on video is no exception to this! Physical examinations of an intimate nature should be conducted outside the view of the camera. The informed consent of the patient is essential. Written consent must be obtained on the approved consent form (there is now a common consent form for both assessment methods). Consent must be sought before the video recording takes place and confirmed after the consultation is over. The patient must understand why the recording is being made, the purposes for which it is being used, who will see it and how long it will remain in existence. There should be no coercion. A well-practised procedure at the reception desk is helpful in obtaining informed consent. Good quality and positive publicity within the practice will help to inform the patients and reduce the number who refuse to give their consent to be videotaped.

There are some patient groups who may find it difficult to give informed consent – for example, the mentally ill, the very ill and non-English-speaking patients. Children and those with learning difficulties are also vulnerable. I recommend that you read the guidelines of the General Medical Council[6] and the Royal College of General Practitioners[7] on consent and confidentiality.

Consultations should be selected wisely

The registrar should present a range of clinical scenarios. New patients or new presentations often provide good opportunities to demonstrate competence, and are much more likely to give enough evidence to pass the MRCGP and gain a merit! Low-challenge consultations should be avoided at all costs, as they are not helpful to assessors of either method. Candidates who submit tapes full of low-challenge consultations often fail.

Further information

The *Blue Book, Conference of Postgraduate Advisers in General Practice Universities of the United Kingdom: Summative Assessment General Practice Training – August 2000* (fourth edition) describes the current rules and regulations, and is updated annually. Copies of the *Blue Book* and further information may be obtained from each deanery's summative assessment office. For information on the MRCGP examination, refer to the RCGP website, which is regularly updated. The Examination Department is also very helpful.

References

1   Pendleton D, Schofield T, Tate P and Havelock P (1984) *The Consultation: an Approach to Learning and Teaching*. Oxford University Press, Oxford.

2   Skelton J, Field SJ, Hammond P and Wiskin C (1999) *Watching You, Watching Me... Consulting Skills and Summative Assessment in General Practice* (2e). Radcliffe Medical Press, Oxford.

3   Skelton J, Field SJ, Wiskin C and Tate P (1998) *Those Things You Say... Consulting Skills and the MRCGP Examination*. Radcliffe Medical Press, Oxford.

4   Tate P (2001) *The Doctor's Communication Handbook* (3e). Radcliffe Medical Press, Oxford.

5   Neighbour R (1987) *The Inner Consultation*. Kluwer Academic Publications, London.

6   General Medical Council (1994) *Further Guidance on the Use of Video-Recordings. Report of the Committee on Standards of Professional Conduct and on Medical Ethics*. General Medical Council, London.

7   Royal College of General Practitioners (1993) *The Use of Video Recording of General Practice Consultations for Teaching, Learning and Assessment: the Importance of Ethical Considerations*. Royal College of General Practitioners, London.

20

Simulated surgeries for summative assessment

Justin Allen and Alison Evans

Although the title of the workshop was *Running Simulated Surgery in Your Own Deanery*, in true adult education style the participants – who just about outnumbered the conveners – were asked what issues they wished to discuss. In a brainstorming session it was decided to discuss in the following topics:

- the effect on registrars and their training programmes of introducing simulated patient assessment
- the effect on training practices (in particular the use of video) of consulting skills training
- the effect of the introduction of the MRCGP
- the practicalities of registrars availing themselves of simulated surgeries
- the knock-on value of having a simulated patient resource.

At the time of the workshop, 32 registrars had been through the system in South Trent and 40 registrars in Yorkshire. Four had been referred for a second simulated surgery, and so far all of them had passed.

In both deaneries it was reported that GP registrars were very positive, and in fact we have been surprised at the level of uptake. It is voluntary in both deaneries at present, but the vast majority of registrars are opting to do it and talking of waiting to do the MRCGP at a later date in their training. The ease of conducting summative assessment and the rapidity with which the result is obtained seem to be key features in this.

Much to everyone's surprise, so far training practices have responded well in that they can actually return to using video for true training purposes, and not merely for the construction of tapes for summative assessment.

The effect of the MRCGP is difficult to evaluate. Certainly some directors and advisers have been holding back on developing simulated surgeries because they feel that their registrars will opt for the MRCGP. However, it was pointed out that there is now a significant pressure to increase the availability of simulated patient assessment in the membership examination.

The three possible methods of making simulated patient assessment available were described. The first is that, with the approval of the director of the deanery concerned, a registrar may simply apply and be directed to the nearest simulated surgery assessment centre, come for the simulated patient assessment and receive their results. This has already had significant uptake in that about 10 of the GP registrars who have so far undertaken simulated surgery have been from outside the two prime deaneries. The deanery concerned will be billed for £150 and will also have to find travel and subsistence costs.

The second method would be for full simulated surgeries to be arranged in deaneries by either the Yorkshire or the South Trent simulated patient teams. This was something that was done extensively during the development phase, but so far has not been arranged. The advantage for GP registrars is that they do not have to travel and they are in relatively familiar surroundings. The deaneries concerned would have to finance the running of a simulated surgery for eight candidate doctors, find suitable premises, and also provide the travel and subsistence costs for the simulator team, which would have to be done by individual negotiation.

Finally, we discussed the transfer of simulated surgery to a deanery, and Alison Evans described how the Yorkshire team had developed their expertise through joint workshops with the Leicester team and then developing their own simulator expertise. This is certainly a possibility that can be explored with any interested deanery. The whole process would take about 12 to 18 months, and the key person to be identified is a simulator co-ordinator.

We had little time in which to discuss the knock-on value. Our experience is that simulated patients in this type of organisation are an extremely valuable teaching resource both for the half-day release course and for trainer education and a number of other applications.

21

Looking after registrars with difficulties: the role of advanced training practices

Maureen Crawford

Introduction

Over the past three years, approximately 50 general practice registrars per year have failed one or more elements of summative assessment in the UK. Of these, perhaps 40 have applied for and been granted extended training. Recent changes in the summative assessment protocols which allow a resubmission of evidence within the standard training time may reduce the number of registrars seeking extensions, but not the number failing. Changes resulting from the MADEL transfer also allow for extensions to training when problems are recognised at any time during the training period before formal failure.

Failure causes distress and loss of self-esteem to the registrar and also, to a lesser extent, to the trainer. Expense to the Director of Postgraduate General Practice Education's budget is incurred by those who need further training. It is arguable that this situation may indicate 'system failure' rather than just failure of individual registrars, particularly if the first indication of problems was a failure in summative assessment.

Helping general practice registrars with problems

The issue of helping registrars with problems, specifically those who had failed summative assessment, was identified by a group of Associate Advisers who had worked together on trainer development at the 1999 UKCRA Conference. As a result, two events were planned: first, a workshop for trainers and others working in this field to be held in Stratford on 19 and 20 October

1999, and secondly, a meeting of Associate Advisers at the Royal College of General Practitioners in London on 24 November 1999.

A total of 30 participants met at Stratford with the aims of sharing experiences, identifying issues to be addressed, starting to generate solutions and devising a consensus statement for consideration nationally. Three small groups brainstormed needs, and the results were used to set up a number of workshops, of which each group chose two.

One of the most enlightening sessions looked at the case histories of 18 registrars who had encountered problems (half of that year's 'failed' cohort). From this session the following themes emerged.

Issues relating to selection

Issues relating to unsatisfactory performance in the past

In many cases there was a history of problems that had been noticed but not acted upon earlier in the doctor's career. The nature of the hospital component of training, with changes of supervisor (or even hospital trust) every six months or even more often allowed SHOs to be given the 'benefit of the doubt' instead of the help that they needed.

Issues relating to the needs of training practices

- This is often much more challenging and time-consuming than 'standard' training. Registrars who have encountered problems need more pastoral care and more supervision (sometimes substantially more, and occasionally even case-by-case debriefing). Trainers can feel isolated and inadequately supported.
- There is a need for extra resources.
- There is a need for support for the trainer who realises that their registrar is showing early warning signs of failing some aspect of summative assessment. Trainers have a strong sense of commitment to helping their registrar pass assessments, and can become uncertain about both their role and where to turn if difficulties are encountered.

Issues relating to the needs of the registrar

- Individual needs assessment and education plan.
- Regular formative assessment.
- The need for an 'advocate' who looks after the needs of the registrar and who is divorced from the assessment process.
- Health problems, including serious mental health problems. Some worrying outcomes for both patients and doctors were reported, including the

tragic suicide of a young registrar who had been advised by her psychiatrist not to reveal her illness as it might damage her career.

The meeting of advisers developed these themes further. The rest of this chapter is distilled from the two meetings.

Prevention and early diagnosis of problems

There seemed to be inextricable links between 'prevention' in terms of selection of registrars and early diagnosis of problems, and dealing with those registrars who have already failed one or more elements of summative assessment. Consequently, the work of both groups crossed these boundaries. Some of the issues and recommendations relate to skills or mechanisms that are needed by all trainers – for example, early diagnosis of problems. Others relate to the special needs of trainers with registrars who have identified problems.

Selection

The MADEL transfer of funding has made this a national issue, which is already the subject of scrutiny under the initiative of Steve Field. The group's recommendations have been incorporated into his work. They included the following:

- the need for an agreed entry standard using a valid and reliable screening tool (MCQ and/or psychometric tests)
- appropriate information sharing, including knowledge of earlier assessments. References should be standardised and should include one from the most recent employer
- interviews should be structured using trained interviewers and complying with employment law. A course for interviewers is planned for autumn 2000
- careful scrutiny of curricula vitae, especially unexplained gaps
- use of a health questionnaire before appointment, with access to an occupational health service where appropriate.

Early identification of difficulty

There is a need for a transparent valid formative system with clear two-way links to the training system. The first three months are vital. This arrangement might be amenable to development nationally. It is important that identification of difficulty triggers urgent action involving the registrar, trainer, course organiser and/or adviser. An educational plan should be agreed, including a clear agreement on monitoring (by whom and when).

Training for registrars with problems

This should include the following:

- identification of suitable ('advanced'?) training practices
- training and support for such practices.

The qualities, needs and experiences of such practices will be examined in more detail below.

Advanced training practices

Features of such practices include willingness to undertake the work and undergo relevant training.

- It is helpful to have two trainers in the practice.
- They should have a good track record with previous registrars and at re-accreditation visits.
- It is helpful to have a geographical spread of available practices.
- Physical requirements such as space need to be taken into consideration.
- They may possess special skills, especially video teaching.

There is no agreed mechanism for allowing extra resources to go to the practice (if needed). Two regional methods of providing such training were reported. The first was in the West Midlands region. A cohort of training practices with status as 'advanced training practices' has been identified. These have special skills, support from a designated course organiser, and are paid an honorarium. One such individual, Merlyn Wilcox, described his experiences at Stratford. Problems included time, patient issues (ethics, consent and availability of trainer) and funding. This reinforced the fact that this type of training is a time-consuming process with implications for all of the partners, staff and patients in the practice. It was sometimes necessary to pay for locum help. Merlyn Wilcox also emphasised the satisfying end result of helping an initially hurt and confused registrar to improve his consulting skills sufficiently to pass summative assessment and regain his confidence.

The second regional method reported was in Northern Ireland, where there are identified advanced training practices with a dual role, combining availability to help registrars with problems and the provision of extended training for a pilot scheme that allows 18 months in practice (instead of the usual 12).

Occupational health service

There is general agreement that all doctors, including registrars, should have access to occupational health services. As far as possible, 'fitness to practise' decisions should be distinct from help for the doctor with difficulties. It is important that there is access to confidential counselling – with the obvious proviso of complying with the duty to protect the public, as outlined by the General Medical Council.

Confidential enquiry

Failing summative assessment is a major blow both to the registrar and to the training practice. It may reflect failure(s) in the system, and it would be helpful to have a mechanism for confidential enquiry into each failure, to enable further patterns and learning points to emerge.

National working group

There has been unanimous support for a working group to examine all issues where it would be useful to standardise practice – for example, funding to support practices with a registrar who has problems. Following discussion among those present at this session, it was agreed that this was a suitable role for a subgroup of the newly formed UKCRA. Maureen Crawford agreed to take this forward, and several other individuals volunteered their help.

Further information

For further information and offers of help contact Maureen Crawford NICPMDE, 5 Annadale Ave, Belfast BT7 3JH (Tel 028 90492731).

Part 7

Continuing professional development

Continuing professional development (CPD) is a process of lifelong learning for all individuals and teams. It should reflect the needs of patients and deliver the desired health outcomes and the healthcare priorities of the NHS.

CPD is one of the core components of clinical governance, and it is crucial to the goal of improving the quality of care for our patients. Active participation in CPD will also play a central role in the revalidation of doctors and the re-registration of healthcare professionals by their professional regulatory bodies.

CPD is most effective when it is planned. This means that there should be a reason for doing the CPD, the method of learning should be identified, and there should be some form of follow-up subsequently. It is also important that the aspirations of the individual, the needs of the team and the needs of patients are balanced. In addition, CPD should be integrated into the usual activities of the primary healthcare team. Individuals should integrate their learning with that of other team members whenever it is appropriate to do so.

In this part of the GP jigsaw, leading authorities on CPD give practical advice and discuss both the future of CPD and the pivotal role of GP tutors in managing the change to a culture of lifelong learning in primary care.

22

The future of CPD in primary care: a personal view

Steve Field

Introduction

The maelstrom of activity surrounding CPD in primary care began in 1990 when the 'new contract' was imposed on general practitioners. At the eye of the storm was the Postgraduate Education Allowance (PGEA), which changed the face of continuing medical education by introducing an inducement for GPs to attend meetings in order to accumulate credits towards their allowance. While this had the effect of increasing the number of meetings and courses available to GPs, it also had the unintended effect of rewarding attendance at events (often of dubious educational quality), rather than recognising the importance of personal study and reflective learning. The time is ripe for change.

My vision of CPD is a scenario where all members of the primary health-care team are actively involved in the process of lifelong learning. I believe that we all want to contribute to improving the health of our patients, and that effective education and training are vital in achieving this. It also does not matter how one learns, but it needs to be planned. There needs to be a change in the culture of learning in primary care to enable more effective multiprofessional learning in order to improve the quality of the healthcare that is provided.

A brief history lesson

CPD is a relatively new concept in general practice in the UK. The basic premise has long been that medical schools produced safe doctors who knew enough to get through to retirement! In 1944, the Goodenough Committee[1] stated that 'one of the gravest disadvantages of present-day general practice is that most GPs have neither the time nor opportunity for postgraduate study'. The proposed solution was that courses should be designed for GPs. In 1952, the College of General Practitioners (later to become the Royal College of General Practitioners, or RCGP) was established. Since its first meeting, it has pursued a relentless campaign to raise the profile of CPD. It has lobbied politically, encouraged and supported courses and developed its Membership and Fellowship by assessment procedures and many quality initiatives, including the Accredited Professional Development programme.

The introduction of the PGEA system in 1990 caused controversy, and has continued to be the subject of much debate and criticism. It replaced an even more inadequate system of seniority awards and 'Section 63' payments. An opportunity was missed to introduce more effective arrangements for CPD because of the sensitivity of the 'new contract' and a political compromise to ensure its introduction. PGEA is limited to general practice principals. It disenfranchises the numerous non-principals in the UK. It is also mainly uniprofessional in its focus, barely involving the participation of other members of the primary healthcare team, who have separate professional development systems which are funded independently. The PGEA system allows general practitioners to earn part of their income by mainly attending PGEA-accredited meetings of their choice without having to identify their educational needs. The Chief Medical Officer's (CMO's) review criticised the PGEA system for failing to demonstrate any convincing benefits for patient care. At a local level the PGEA and medical audit systems have developed independently of each other.[1-3] This has resulted in missed opportunities for improving the quality of healthcare.

In order to develop CPD, the Directors of Postgraduate General Practice Education (DPGPE), who are responsible for the accreditation of the PGEA systems in their own deaneries, have adapted the accreditation procedures to encourage personal and reflective learning. This has resulted in many exciting initiatives built on adult learning principles, such as personal learning plans, mentoring schemes and portfolio-based learning. The uptake of these initiatives is voluntary, with the majority of PGEA activity still being unplanned and not based on the individual's learning needs.

Seminal documents on CPD in primary care include the 1997 White Paper, *The NHS: Modern, Dependable*, the Chief Medical Officer's review of continuing professional development in general practice,[4] the consultative document, *A First-Class Service* and the two Standing Committee on Postgraduate Medical Education (SCOPME) papers on the education of GP non-principals,[5] and mentoring.[6]

The CMO's report on CPD and the consultative document, *A First-Class Service*, suggest that in the 'new NHS' most of the work on CPD and clinical governance will take place in GPs' surgeries, pharmacies, dental surgeries, optometrists' shops, etc. The NHS Executive has formed a working party to implement their recommendations. The purpose of the review is to help primary care meet the challenge of changes in the structure and delivery of patient care, such as the development of primary care groups (PCGs) and primary care trusts (PCTs). It aimed to encourage more reflection on practice and learning needs, including more forward planning, and to make the educational methods used in practice more effective. It should signal the end of the much maligned postgraduate educational allowance system and herald the beginning of a more integrated system of education with a focus on the multiprofessional primary healthcare team.

Educational infrastructures at practice level

Supportive educational infrastructures for clinical governance and CPD are required at practice level to provide a positive force for improving patient care. I propose that each practice should form a Clinical Governance and CPD Committee. This should be a multidisciplinary group, and it should include all staff – medical, nursing and administrative – including locums, retainer doctors and other GP non-principals. There should be a CPD lead for all staff groups, who should contribute to the development of individuals and the whole practice. Each member of staff should have a Personal and Professional Development Plan (PPDP) which reflects the practice service development plan as well as external influences from a PCG/PCT and health authority level. The practice should also appoint a clinical governance lead, who would be responsible for clinical audit and clinical standards, and have input into the PPDPs and the practice service development plans. The committee would require administrative support (e.g. audit and education secretaries). It would have responsibility for co-ordinating CPD, audit, research and clinical standards. In future, most educational activity will revolve around the practice and the PCG/PCT. External facilitation should be available at a PCG/PCT level, but it is recognised that there are many different ways of learning and that these should be encouraged. The responsibility for approving the practice's PPDPs would fall on the PCG/PCT's clinical governance lead supported by the GP tutors.

Educational infrastructures at PCG/PCT level

Clinical governance leads are typically PCG board members, and clinical governance should remain a director-level function in PCTs. The PCG/PCT should also have a clinical governance and CPD subcommittee, which might include the clinical governance lead, a GP tutor, a nurse tutor and a managerial tutor (for 'tutor', one could read 'educational facilitator'). Administrative support would be required based on a local needs assessment exercise. The committee would look at the needs of the wider PCG and influence the wider personal and practice professional development plans at the lower tier. Under the new proposals recommended in the CMO's review of CPD, the health authority would have final responsibility for endorsing the PPDPs. I recommend that this responsibility should be devolved to the clinical governance lead of the PCG, with advice from the deanery organisation. The health authority could performance-monitor the process as part of their general performance-monitoring role for the PCG.

The educational facilitating role should be undertaken by the professional tutors or educational facilitators (e.g. the GP tutor), with advice and support from the deanery structure. The existing GP tutor networks have proved to be highly successful in developing the education of general practitioners, and have recently moved towards more of a facilitating and mentoring role for individual doctors. This should be encouraged. Nationally, we have been discussing the human resource requirements for PCG/PCTs to meet both CPD needs and the likely requirements of revalidation. It is possible that ten sessions of GP tutor time for every 50 GPs may be required.

A successful CPD and clinical governance subcommittee will ensure that quality improvement processes are in place. It will work with other PCG/PCTs, the health authority, the National Institute for Clinical Excellence (NICE), the Commission for Health Improvement (CHI), etc. to ensure that evidence-supported medicine becomes part of the culture in the PCG/PCT. It will aid dissemination of good practice and guidelines, and it will also provide a framework for sharing lessons learned from patients' suggestions and complaints. The prevention and early detection of poor performance will also be the responsibility of the committee. The GP tutor will have a key role in supporting the practitioners who are identified as requiring educational support, working closely with the wider deanery educational team.

The role of health authorities

Health authorities have an important role to play in the development of the PCG/PCTs, in particular in organisational development and ensuring that there is adequate funding for education and training. The health authority should be encouraged to work closely with the local medical committees (LMCs) to achieve effective functioning of the PCG/PCTs. The health authorities should also work closely with the deanery educational structures with regard to the gradual transfer of the PGEA to the new PPDP system. A partnership will ensure that the CMO's review is implemented without the discomfiture that was experienced with the introduction of the PGEA system. The health authority should monitor the programme to ensure that at all levels the development plans reflect their Health Improvement Programme (HImP) and the national frameworks, but should also acknowledge the need for practices and PCG/PCTs to develop their own style and identity. The deanery GP education structure role is to provide educational advice to the PCG/PCT clinical governance lead and health authority, and to provide independent educational support for the GPs via its GP tutor networks.

The Personal Development Plan (PDP)

The bedrock of the recommendations is the Personal Development Plan (PDP). Because of the emphasis placed on this plan by the *First-Class Service* document, it has become the cornerstone of proposals for development of CPD, in both primary and secondary care. The PDP will be an annual plan agreed with 'an appropriate person'. Figure 22.1 is a pictorial representation of how I believe PDPs fit into the system. Each person working in the NHS should have a PDP that reflects the needs of the practice, but which of course will not be exactly the same as the Practice Professional Development Plan

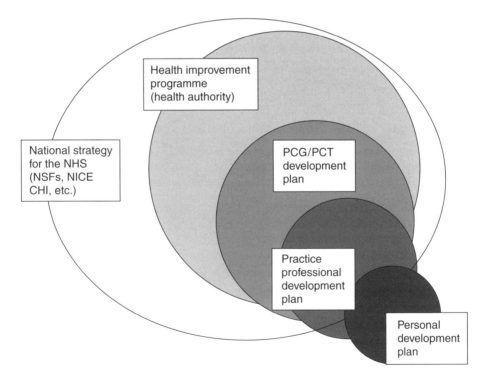

Figure 22.1: The relationship between development plans.[7]

(PPDP), because each person has their own individual needs which require support. The PPDP will fit into the PCG/PCT's development plan, which should reflect the needs identified in the local HImP. The national agenda, including National Service Frameworks, will obviously have an effect on the whole system.

The Practice Professional Development Plan (PPDP)

The PPDP is a record of the overall plans for the development of the team and all of the individuals within it. It should draw on practice clinical audit findings and local needs assessment, and should involve users and carers. It will describe how needs are to be met and include sections on quality control, dissemination of learning outcomes and a review of the previous year's plan. Clinical governance leads will look at the PPDPs to ensure that the needs of the individual, practice, PCG/PCT, NHS and the patients are balanced.

The role of GP tutors

GP tutors will have an important role to play in supporting the development of the PDP at the individual practice and PCG/PCT levels. They are a valuable resource, and have started to take on the challenge. They are well placed to facilitate a change in the culture and help to create an environment that is conducive to effective lifelong learning and continuing professional development. They have leadership at a local level as well as being able to support the provision of educational activities and act as a facilitator and mentor. In the short term, they should work closely with their tutor colleagues in the other professional groups to provide a more co-ordinated system of CPD in their localities. However, I believe that the title 'GP tutor' is out of date, and that we should move quickly to a system where 'primary care tutors' support CPD in the PCG/PCTs, with the only criterion being that they should have the appropriate skills for the role, rather than being selected because they belong to a particular staff group.

And finally...

I believe that investment in lifelong learning is an investment in quality. The GP tutor network is a supportive facility that is developing to meet the needs of general practitioners and other primary care staff to support the development of PDPs, PPDPs, lifelong learning and reflective practice skills. Investment in teambuilding and in leadership courses will also be needed to support the development of primary care. None of this will happen without a political commitment to bring about its realisation.

References

1   Periera Gray D (1992) *The Continuing Education Story Forty Years On. The Story of the First Forty Years of the Royal College of General Practitioners*. Royal College of General Practitioners, London.

2   Houghton PG (1996) Linking clinical audit and continuing medical education. A report from the National Primary Care Audit Meeting. *Audit Trends*. **4**: 1–2.

3   Primary Health Care Clinical Audit Working Group of the Clinical Outcomes Group (1995) *Clinical Audit in Primary Health Care*. Department of Health, London.

4   Department of Health (1998) *A Review of Continuing Professional Development in General Practice. Report by the Chief Medical Officer*. Department of Health, London.

5   Standing Committee on Postgraduate Medical and Dental Education (1998) *The Educational Needs of General Practice Non-Principals*. Standing Committee on Postgraduate Medical and Dental Education, London.

6   Standing Committee on Postgraduate Medical and Dental Education (1998) *An Enquiry into Mentoring, Supporting Doctors and Dentists at Work*. Standing Committee on Postgraduate Medical and Dental Education, London.

7   Field SJ (1999) The future of continuing professional development in primary care. *Educ Gen Pract*. **10**: 339–41.

23

The National Association of GP Tutors' view of the future role of the GP tutor in CPD, revalidation and fitness to practise

Malcolm Valentine

Introduction

The National Association of GP Tutors (NAGPT) was established as a professional body for GP tutors in 1993. It is a 'subset' of UKCRA.

The past decade has seen an accelerated rate of change in the organisation and delivery of healthcare in the UK. Primary care has perhaps been the most exposed element of the UK healthcare system. 1990 saw the advent of the Postgraduate Education Allowance (PGEA) regulations, which we seem to be stuck with, as well as the major changes brought about by GP fundholding. Political change in the latter part of the decade saw the removal of GP fundholding as part of wide-ranging reorganisation involving the introduction of practice groupings into primary care groups and their equivalents in the devolved UK countries.

The introduction of clinical governance, performance assessment and the imminent introduction of revalidation will all have increasing effects in determining the future complexion of primary care delivery. Revalidation will necessitate the *explicit* demonstration of fitness to practise, including continuing appraisal and lifelong learning by every practitioner maintaining registration with the General Medical Council (GMC).

Inevitably, new systems of managed continuing professional development (CPD) will be required to underpin these changes. The NAGPT believes that the current network of GP tutors is well placed, under the direction of the Directors of Postgraduate GP Education (DPGPEs), to evolve into a network of primary care tutors. Utilising appropriate tools and methodologies, and with respect for colleagues as mutual adult learners, primary care tutors have a vital role in conducting formative appraisal and facilitated professional development, and ensuring that GPs can fulfil the requirements of revalidation when they arise.

The NAGPT proposals are more fully described in *Vision 2000 – Managed CPD in the New NHS*, which was published in February 2000 and is available from the NAGPT office (email: nagpt@btinternet.com).

To cover the future role of the GP tutor in CPD, revalidation and fitness to practise in one workshop is a tall order. It was decided to engage workshop participants in debate before then giving the NAGPT view. This article therefore summarises the views of participants as well as giving the views of the NAGPT.

A debate: what is the UKCRA view of the future role of the GP tutor in CPD, revalidation and fitness to practise?

The following issues were raised by participants at the UKCRA conference workshop.

1 The GP tutor in CPD:
   • has a vital role in supporting PDPs, PPDPs and working with practices
   • needs to be part of 'learning groups'
   • needs to incorporate National Service Framework (NSF)/National Institute for Clinical Excellence (NICE) priorities into their activities
   • needs to manage CPD, so requires business planning skills and appropriate funding
   • needs to change their role (and possibly title) to CPD co-ordinator
   • may have to forgo their one-to-one role
   • may evolve into a two-tier network (i.e. PCG-based and locality-based)
   • needs to attain appropriate skills for their task
   • needs proper planning, clear strategy and a properly managed structure
   • needs clear lines of responsibility and support
   • needs strong *national* leadership.
2 The GP tutor in revalidation:
   • should be a facilitator rather than a policeman
   • appraisal should be educational – it does not include 'signing off'
   • clinical governance groups undertake practice accreditation. The GP tutor may need to handle collateral damage
   • there is an urgent need for extra GP tutor capacity *now*
   • needs to ensure that individuals produce a satisfactory portfolio

- will need to offer a communication skills assessment service
- GP trainers are an as yet untapped resource
- terms and conditions may need to be changed to allow GP tutors to be paid a 'proper' salary
- there is an overarching need to protect the GP work-force
- there is a need for a clear system – UK-wide
- there is a need to develop 'Educational Centres', especially for non-principals.

3   The GP tutor in fitness to practise:
- local remediation will be costly, and is currently based on dubious methodology
- there are difficulties when faced with resistance to intervention
- there are concerns about litigation and legal challenge
- there is a danger of being sucked into time-intensive, resource-intensive, mentally draining personal mentoring
- there is a need to establish funding, protected time, support and suitable personnel
- it may be necessary to charge individuals for the 'whole package'.

The NAGPT response

CPD is 'a process of lifelong learning for all individuals and teams which enables professionals to expand and fulfil their potential and which also meets the needs of patients and delivers the healthcare priorities of the NHS'.[1] This definition adequately summarises the mutual issues of personal need, organisational need and the imperative of enhanced patient care.

Knowledge and learning

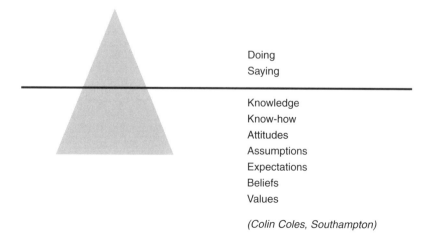

Doing
Saying

Knowledge
Know-how
Attitudes
Assumptions
Expectations
Beliefs
Values

(Colin Coles, Southampton)

Professor Colin Coles from Southampton has presented this concept on a number of occasions. In looking at what is essentially the question of how to manage a system of continuing medical education, it is essential to bear in mind what that system is trying to achieve. The primary purpose is to motivate adult learners towards enhanced knowledge, skills and consequently quality of care. Summative approaches will inevitably do little more than manipulate the issues above the line. However, what is really important is what lies beneath the line.

The traditional GPT role – *visible*

This role includes the following elements:

- a purveyor of educational meetings
- a useful pair of hands in the PGEA approvals business
- a variable facilitation/resource function.

This is the traditional role of the GP tutor, as it has been perceived by many. It represents a narrow view of a cohort of educators who have evolved considerably, both personally and as a network. This evolution has accelerated considerably over the past three years.

The traditional GPT role – *hidden*

This role includes the following elements:

- a highly skilled group
- wide involvement in an extended range of promoted posts and activities
- resourceful, independent, self-reliant and creative
- a strong orientation to adult learning models (intentional or intuitive) restrained by current practices
- wide involvement in change management
- strong leadership potential.

In fact, this is a more accurate representation of the role of the GP tutor. In the absence of a clear, nationally managed structure, they have in many cases sought out the most productive way to utilise considerable expertise and talent.

The primary care tutor's future role in CPD

- Motivating change requires the input of a wise peer who is non-judgemental. Self-directed learning occurs when people take part in planning their own

learning, in deciding what and how to learn and, when they have a chance to do so, to reflect upon the benefits of that learning.
- It requires resourcing and facilitation, commitment to change and appropriate tools.

(Self Directed Learning for GPs, Conclusions, Study Day, April 1998)

In presenting a view of the future, the first point is that the title and function of the appointment have to change. The term 'primary care tutor' suggests a wider remit. Restating the educational imperative is vital. Ideally the primary care network must develop into empowered, self-directed adult learners. The primary care tutor's role is to effect and manage this.

The primary care tutor as a manager of CPD

This role includes the following elements:

- some direct appraisal
- direct appraisals by others
- educational support, including materials (e.g. desktop portfolio), new ideas, public health input, etc.
- accreditation and certification (to keep the employers happy)
- a conduit for guidelines and audit
- strategic developments (e.g. revalidation, organisational change)
- networking and resource finding
- educational cultural development.

(see NAGPT Vision 2000: Managed CPD in the New NHS)[2]

These points start to develop the notion of the primary care tutor as a manager of CPD. It is interesting to note that these qualities also represent those of a 'manager of change' within the primary care system. Extending the primary care tutor's role to supporting the implementation of national strategies could enhance and accelerate such changes.

The future role of the primary care tutor – terms

These are as follows:

- one tutor for approximately 50 GPs, plus staff, plus individuals with a developmental role, plus new service developments
- GP tutor – minimum two-session appointment for a cohort of 50 GPs, assisted by educational leads and/or mentors, with input from clinical governance lead (as recommended by *Vision 2000*)

- dual accountability to the PCG and to the Director of Postgraduate GP Education
- funded via MADEL – essential to retain strategic educational/developmental network
- future opportunities (e.g. revalidation).

Surprisingly, the terms and conditions for the primary care tutor are still as unclear as ever. There is huge regional variation in both workload and expectation. This is directly influenced by the lack of an agreed national strategy or role. It really is a matter of urgency for these issues to be addressed, otherwise the notion of a clearly defined national network may fail to materialise.

The primary care tutor 'habitat' (1)

This has the following characteristics:

- continues to interact closely with the Director network
- quality assurance development groups (happening already)
- district-wide
- multi-representative
- remit is continuous improvement
- co-ordinates clinical governance and guideline development
- mutual support among professional groups and organisational structures
- co-ordinates delivery of all education and training
- consistency
- health information strategy
- co-ordinates development bids
- informs new educational ventures.

The NAGPT has described clearly how the primary care tutor may develop in its publication *Vision 2000: Managed CPD in the New NHS*. In this booklet we examined the remit that local 'quality development groups' might have. These represent an efficient way of bringing together all of those involved in quality assurance activities and allowing the primary care tutor to develop a lead role in ensuring the professional development of individuals to support such issues.

The primary care tutor 'habitat' (2)

This has the following characteristics:

- integrates closely with clinical governance lead
- works closely with educational lead

- works with RCGP faculty and/or RCGP accreditation systems
- works with LMC representative to ensure conformity with terms and conditions.

In a properly managed system, the primary care tutor will have to be accountable in a number of different ways. In order to benefit from the support of the 'postgraduate family', NAGPT strongly argues that the tutor network should remain within the line management of the directors' network. The links above illustrate other obvious, key people. These roles are described more specifically in *Vision 2000*.

The primary care tutor and revalidation (1)

This includes the following:

- GMC consultation document (May 2000)
- construction of curriculum vitae and description of work
- good medical practice for GPs
- good clinical care
- maintaining good clinical practice
- working with colleagues
- relationship with patients
- teaching and training
- probity
- health.

The NAGPT contends that primary care tutors will play a critical role in the implementation of revalidation. General practice has consistently come out in favour of a revalidation process, and needs to be supported in ensuring that the process becomes successful and meaningful. The GMC consultation document has now been circulated, and the final complexion of revalidation procedures will become apparent by the end of the year.

The primary care tutor and revalidation (2)

This includes the following:

- a review of complaints
- a structured critical incident analysis
- a description of clinical service and adverse service conditions
- an action plan
- the agreed outcome of the appraisal
- a time-frame

- a signed statement from the appraiser
- no surprises.

Revalidation will have substantial (and many as yet unpredictable) effects. The task is massive. There are in excess of 40 000 doctors working in primary care. The work required to ensure success in producing the necessary material will demand high-quality support and strong national leadership. The profession will not take kindly to unpleasant surprises.

The primary care tutor and revalidation (3)

This includes the following:

- appraisal
- it should be *formative* – *performance* achieves little in 'autonomous' professional groups (British Association of Medical Managers, *Appraisal in Action*)
- but:
  (i) how often?
  (ii) by primary care tutor or educational lead or someone else?
  (iii) standardised tools and methodology?
- resources?
- it should result in a spiral of supported enhancement of individual professional development.

Appraisal is now well described – even in medical circles. An excellent recent publication which describes the processes of performance and developmental appraisal very clearly is *Appraisal in Action*,[3] which is available from the British Association of Medical Managers. It is essential that skilled appraisal systems are developed which encompass the professional development of individuals, and do not just fulfill performance targets.

The primary care tutor and revalidation (4)

The process:

- needs to be described and reasonably uniform across the UK
- integrates national processes with regional priorities, incorporates personal/practice/group methodologies, and involves multiprofessional development.

The NAGPT:

- is developing a framework which provides a model for the whole process
- uses simple/effective systems, tools, pro forma

- has a desktop computer portfolio which is essential, easily understood, implementable and can evolve (actionable first step).

The NAGPT suggests the need for processes to be reasonably uniform across the UK. We strongly support the GMC as a UK-wide organisation. There must be freedom of movement within the UK which is not jeopardised by parochial ideas and solutions with low transferability elsewhere. The NAGPT believes that it can go on to contribute much to the evolving debate and to assist in the development of the necessary tools and methodologies.

The primary care tutor and fitness to practise

Supporting Doctors, Protecting Patients[4]

- This is due to be resurrected in the autumn.
- Are 'Gulags' appropriate when it is usually the system that has failed? Are they even remotely educationally valid?

'Retraining'

- This is time- and resource-intensive, and individually taxing.
- There is little evidence that GP tutors will have the requisite skills (but also little evidence that anyone else does).

Should we accept the summative nature of revalidation and prepare for the casualties and collateral damage?

This is a contentious issue which requires further debate. The purported 'retraining centres' are invalid, especially in the face of a resistant learner. The time and resource implications have already been mentioned. The skill base simply does not exist at present. The NAGPT has debated this issue at length. Whilst it is always optimistic and supportive of fellow professionals, the role of the primary care tutor may be to provide that support to those who are affected by the collateral damage which may result from GPs who are deemed unfit to practise.

Conclusion

The NAGPT has lobbied hard over the past six years to raise the profile of the GP tutor. We have given our view of how this role can be devolved to someone with more holistic responsibilities within the primary care arena. The NAGPT has produced carefully considered material in an attempt to define a system for 'managed CPD', and will continue to develop tools to support these changes.

The role of the primary care tutor needs to be agreed *now*. The human and infrastructure resourcing needs to be agreed upon and then secured. These matters are becoming an imperative. Around 40 000 practitioners will have high expectations that the postgraduate structures can deliver.

References

1   Chief Medical Officer (1998) *A Review of Continuing Professional Development in General Practice*. Department of Health, London.

2   Valentine M and Howard J (2000) *Vision 2000: Managed CPD in the New NHS*. National Association of GP Tutors UK, Manchester.

3   Simpson J and Haines S (1999) *Appraisal in Action*. British Association of Medical Managers, Stockport. www.bamm.co.uk

4   Chief Medical Officer (1999) *Supporting Doctors, Protecting Patients. A consultation paper*. Department of Health, London.

Further reading

GP Learning (2000) *Doctors' Desktop Portfolio*. www.gplearning.com

Spencer-Jones R (1998) Self-directed learning: where now? *Educ Gen Prac*. **9**: 498–501.

24

The changing role of the GP tutor

Neil Jackson and Mike Grenville

Historical background

In the North Thames (East) deanery, all GP tutors' contracts expired at the end of March 1999. With the simultaneous advent of primary care groups (PCGs), an opportunity existed to review the role of the GP tutor and to revise the job description and personal specification. A network of multiprofessional/multidisciplinary GP tutors had already been well established by this time under the LIZEI programme (1995–1998). A total of 36 GP tutor sessions were then available and funded through the North Thames (East) Postgraduate Department's MADEL budget. The Department also related to a total of 35 PCGs across seven health authorities covering North Central London, City and East London and Essex.

A review of the role of the GP tutor

Towards the end of 1998 the Director of Postgraduate General Practice Education (DPGPE) and the Deputy DPGPE met with representatives of the GP tutor network to review the role of the GP tutor. Taking into account all continuing medical education (CME) activity at the time, and the Government's agenda for primary care development, including the establishment of PCGs (and eventually primary care trusts or PCTs), it was agreed that the GP tutor's role and function should encompass the following three main areas of activity:

1   the traditional role of the GP tutor in relation to PGEA-generated activities
2   encouraging and facilitating the development of educational initiatives that were established under the LIZEI programme (e.g. self-directed learning groups, mentoring schemes, etc.)
3   a new area of activity to facilitate the process of education and development at organisational, team and healthcare professional levels by attachment

to the 35 PCGs in the North Thames (East) deanery. It was also recognised that each primary care tutor would need to work closely with the PCG clinical governance and education leads.

It was agreed that henceforth the title of the GP tutor should be changed to 'primary care tutor' to reflect all three areas of activity, and to take into account the multiprofessional ethos. On that basis, a revised job description and personal specification were developed, and the Deputy Dean PGPE then proceeded to manage the process of recruiting and appointing a new cohort of primary care tutors, assisted by representatives of the 35 PCGs, LMCs and health authority education boards. To ensure good human resources practice and equal opportunities during the selection and appointment procedures, advice was sought from the Head of Human Resources at Thames Post-graduate Medical and Dental Education (TPMDE), University of London.

Bringing funding streams together

Where possible the Department increased the total number of 36 primary care tutor sessions already established by seizing on additional funding opportunities from health authority education boards and PCGs. This proved successful in a number of cases, and as a result additional tutors were appointed to work specifically from NHS Trust postgraduate centres, or to co-ordinate local networks of primary care tutors attached to PCGs.

A strategic approach to education and training – PCGs and the changing role of the GP tutor

It was recognised that by attaching primary care tutors to PCGs we could provide strategic direction from within the deanery by emphasising through the tutor network the importance of a firm partnership between the three NHS systems (i.e. service provision, education and training and research and development – a 'three-systems' approach). The North Thames (East) Post-graduate GP Department also determined that the future development of the primary care tutor network should be underpinned by a set of core principles, defined as listed below:

- political context
- ownership (by PC tutors, PCGs, etc.)
- partnership (with other organisations, stakeholders, etc.)
- building of existing achievements (post-LIZEI, etc.)

- strategic vision/leadership (from regional office, deanery)
- a multiprofessional/multidisciplinary context
- a multipurpose role (facilitation, support, development, educational provider, etc.)
- locality focus/solutions (various models)
- evaluation
- personal and professional development for each primary care tutor.

Working with PCGs: a practical model

There are various ways in which primary care tutors can work effectively with PCGs. One particular model (*see* Figure 24.1) has emerged in East

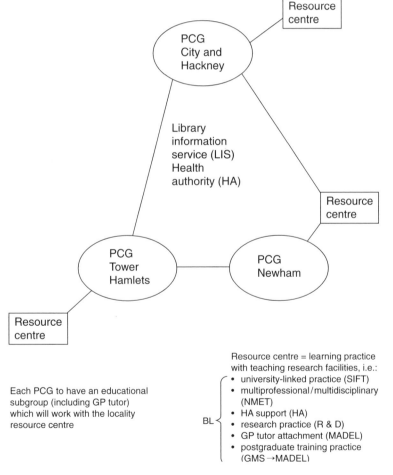

Figure 24.1:   Model of primary care tutors working with PCGs, developed in East London and City Health Authority (ELCHA).

London and City Health Authority (ELCHA), which has three large PCGs each supported by an education resource centre – a post-LIZEI initiative. The model also emphasises the key partnerships between PCGs, health authority, education consortium (CELEC – i.e. City and East London Education Consortium) and the deanery (TPMDE). The importance of bringing together the various funding streams for education and training is also highlighted.

The development of personal development plans and practice/professional development plans – a pilot model

A new facet of GP tutor work has been the facilitation of the production of both practice/professional and personal development plans. Within the North Thames (East) Deanery each PCG is using a different format, although they are all rooted in patients' unmet needs (PUNs) and doctors' educational needs (DENs). The Redbridge and Waltham Forest group has set up a multiprofessional organisation to facilitate this process using a method known as force-field analysis. This enables a whole practice approach to be used for the development of an 'educational plan'. This plan, which is the non-confidential outcome of a confidential process, has to take account of both national and local health improvement programme priorities, as well as any needs that are specific to the practice. All practice plans are then fed into the PCG boards to be used to inform both the commissioning of services and the educational programme for the PCG, both as part of a wider health economy and within its own locality/practice base. Interestingly this project, which is being funded by the Outer London Education Consortium, has met with resistance from only one group of GP practices. The other major triumph has been the acceptance of the non-GP group members as facilitators and the value placed on their input. This process is of itself quite time-consuming – it takes at least three and a half hours to do a proper force-field analysis. The group has also taken time out to learn how to facilitate the process.

The UKCRA workshop (June 2000)

Using the concepts illustrated above, the workshop participants discussed the future role of the GP tutor from the deanery perspective. There was general agreement that the future was uncertain. It is uncertain whether the GP tutors will remain part of the deanery network in three years' time (national guidelines are awaited). It was also felt that the ideal minimum support should be one MADEL session per tutor for deanery business (i.e. GP personal needs) and one PCG/PCT session for practice development. It was also agreed that the PCG/PCT would have its own organisational, educational and developmental needs.

The discussion then focused on the GP tutors' own personal development. The delegates discussed their personal development and job development in the light of the following:

- the amalgamation of education funding streams and the formation of local work-force confederations
- professional reaccreditation/revalidation and the need to address these issues with or for their constituents
- mentorship and support for colleagues
- the role of the postgraduate centre lectures and maintenance skills.

Finally there was a discussion about the selection process that we had used in the North Thames (East) deanery for GP tutors. This is based on a fairly well-defined person specification and job specification with an evaluated structured interview, so that in the event of an appeal it could be shown that there was objectivity with no unfair discrimination.

In conclusion, we felt that we should use the recent work-force publication[1] as an opportunity to work together across professions and deaneries, but we must not throw the baby out with the bath water and lose the good work that GP tutors have already started.

References

1   Department of Health (2000) *A Health Service of all the Talents: Developing the NHS Work-force.* Department of Health, London.

25

Learning as a lever for change: delivering improved care through the activity of GP tutors

Monica McLean, Michael Fisher and Nafsika Alexiadou

Introduction

The project relates to education for general practitioners (GPs) in Shropshire and Staffordshire, a part of the West Midlands deanery. It began in late summer 1999 with the aims of determining the optimal role for a GP tutor based with a primary care group (PCG) and describing a variety of models which, in an acceptable and rewarding environment, could meet the individual learning needs of practitioner, practice and PCG, and consequently demonstrate an improvement in the care of individual patients.'[1]

The role of the GP tutor as a peer who organises educational events for GPs is well established in the two counties. The project aimed to elaborate the role of the GP tutor in a context of increasing pressure on the profession to demonstrate that continuing professional development (CPD) is being taken seriously. The more specific objectives of the project are that GP tutors work with PCGs to facilitate understanding of the nature and implications of current practice and of sharing good practice. A further objective is to determine whether and how GP education and training impact on patient care.

The evaluation of the 'Learning as a Lever to Deliver Change' project

The evaluation of the project[2] was conducted along the principles of formative evaluation, whereby the 'subjects' of the evaluation (in this case the director of the project and six GP tutors) are invited to respond to the findings of the evaluation and to shape it.

The aim was to evaluate the extent to which the project's objectives had been achieved, to explore the significance of the GP tutor role, and to outline and analyse models of GP education and training.

The following methods were used to gather the evidence that has informed this report:

- four meetings with the director of the project to discuss issues and progress
- one group meeting with GP tutors[3]
- taped interviews with six GP tutors
- the responses of GP tutors to a short paper outlining the main issues arising from interviews with them
- telephone interviews with a primary care medical advisor, a director of health policy and public health and a primary care group (PCG) chief executive
- information from national and local policy-related documents
- a literature review charting the relationship between the state and the medical profession since 1945.

Historical and political context

The social and political context of the project is one in which GPs are 'being expected to be more accountable and to demonstrate their competence and adherence to minimum standards of care'.[4] At present, the expectation has become a demand fuelled by what could be referred to as 'moral panic' in the wake of a number of highly publicised misdemeanours by doctors.[5] The main theme running through this paper is the desire of the medical profession to reconcile professional self-regulation with the need to be accountable, and the desirability of this. This section aims to illuminate the present reforms in the light of their political context and historical development with reference to the post-1946 period. Attention is drawn to similarities in the relationship of the state to other public service professionals, particularly teachers.

Professionals, professionalism and the state

During the period 1930–1950, the professions were viewed as a crucial part of the rebuilding of post-war Britain and of the building of the welfare state. The post-war welfare state relied on the professions to generate social definitions of, for example, health and illness, deviance and normality, educational success and failure, and so on. At the same time, the state and the professions agreed on privileges and conditions of service, such as independence of practice.[6]

The economic crisis of the 1970s prompted strong questioning of both the state's ability to pay for its welfare system and the role of professionals.[7] Furthermore, it has been argued that scepticism about professionals and the power they held came both from the political left (concerned that citizen empowerment was being obstructed by professional power) and from the right (concerned about consumer choice).[8] In response, the Conservative government that was elected in 1979 introduced competitive systems and market practices, signalling a change in the position of professionals.

At the same time a process of increasing state control began. The encroachment of the state on different professions varied according to the positions they already held and their current bargaining power. So, for example, through the introduction of the Education Reform Act, including the National Curriculum, teachers lost control over the school curriculum. At the time teachers were portrayed in the media as over-demanding and self-interested, as peddling socialist propaganda and as marginalising parental interest. 'Moral panic' was created about the state of the nation's education, and teachers were soon subjected to a raft of changes that encroached on their traditional freedom to choose what to teach.

The medical profession was less vulnerable to such policies, since the ideal of clinical freedom was preserved in theory and practice until the late 1990s, and doctors were in a far stronger position with regard to negotiating conditions of service. However, the reforms have now caught up with the health service and have challenged the traditional freedom and autonomy of practice. Doctors now face the same barrage of media attacks that teachers did during the 1970s and 1980s.

The main point to be made in this section is that, for public service professionals, autonomy and privilege can always be lost and need to be defended.[9] There is a body of literature which argues that establishing the boundaries of professionalism is an achievement, and that maintaining them takes the form of a struggle with the state.[10] The professions need to negotiate with the state with regard to recognition, licensing, regulated recruitment and monopolistic practice.

Since the National Health Service Act of 1948 the medical professional has been primarily (although not exclusively) a state professional, and medicine has been a field of public employment. Thus the education and training of doctors, pay and work conditions and funding are all a matter of negotiation between the profession and the state. However, the autonomy enjoyed by the medical profession as a result of its historical relationship with the state is far greater than that of other state professions, such as teaching.

The restructuring of public services

The creation of what is widely known as an internal or quasi-market is a feature of most areas of the public sector as a result of reforms that started in the late 1980s. A combination of reduced funding, the introduction of a market structure, devolved accountability at the point of delivery of services, and strong central regulation gave rise to the major components of what is called *new public management* (NPM) in the public sector. We can summarise three main areas of NPM as they were introduced into the NHS, the education sector (primary, secondary and post-compulsory) and to some extent the police.[11]

1 *Efficiency, cost reduction and centralisation.* Reduced budgets were introduced across the public services, and the cost had to be met at the unit level. Budgetary control and responsibility were devolved to institutions, and external audits proliferated for quality control and for providing comparative information on efficiency and effectiveness.
2 *The market.* The market structure in the public services was primarily characterised by competition for services and by increased customer choice.
3 *Managerial approaches.* Central control of the content of activity increased managerial powers within the institutions of the public sector, since it was the manager's responsibility to implement this. Furthermore, a variety of private sector concepts and practices were introduced in the public sector (e.g. 'customer care', total quality management (TQM), portfolios and the practice of franchising of services).

Restructuring and the NHS

Within this framework of NPM, the most important changes for the NHS were introduced in a first wave of reforms during 1991, and they were characterised by the purchaser–provider split, increased management and increased clinical/cost audits.   The most significant change for GPs was the creation of the 'fundholding system'. The result was the creation of what was effectively a two-tier system in primary care, with fundholding GPs able to establish their own contracts with providers and make savings for reinvestment in practice-based services. The British Medical Association (BMA) resisted the scheme, but it became fairly well established, with 50% of the population being cared for by GP fundholders by the end of the experiment.[12]

The second wave of reforms came in with the Labour government in 1997. The White Paper, *The New NHS: Modern, Dependable*, published by the Department of Health in 1997, set out to dismantle the internal market, and signalled changes in the approaches to quality control and audit in health-care. This paper[13] heralded a wide range of changes.

Primary care groups (PCGs)

PCGs, which had been in place since 1 April 1999, replaced the system of 'fundholder' and assumed devolved health authority (HA) functions. Groups of general practices will provide primary healthcare and purchase hospital and community services for approximately 100 000 people in each locality. The governing boards are accountable to HAs, and are now working in partnership in drawing up purchasing plans and agreed targets for improving health and value for money.[14] It should be noted that PCGs would have the option of acquiring trust status and becoming primary care trusts (PCTs). There will be another shift in responsibilities, the implications of which are beyond the scope of this paper. Those who were spoken to in connection with this evaluation generally regard PCGs as 'bottom-up' and facilitative, but consider that there is a tension with the tone and measures emanating 'from the top', especially with regard to clinical governance.

Clinical governance

Clinical governance was introduced in *A First-Class Service: Quality in the New NHS*, published by the Department of Health in 1998, which describes a systematic model for combining clinical judgement with clear national standards known as national service frameworks (NSFs), which were developed to define pathways through primary, secondary and tertiary care.[15] Clinical governance is the mechanism for delivering the NSFs. It was defined in the *First-Class Service* paper as 'a framework through which NHS organisations are accountable for continuously improving the quality of their services and safeguarding high standards of care by creating an environment in which excellence in clinical care will flourish'. Harrison and Ahmad (2000) point out that 'this anodyne formulation masks a significant challenge to clinical autonomy as previously practised.'

National Institute for Clinical Excellence (NICE)

NICE will make recommendations to government about cost-effectiveness and clinical and service guidelines and models. These recommendations will be based on the current evidence as evaluated by NICE. The recommendations will, within the framework of clinical governance, become a professional obligation.

Commission for Health Improvement (CHI)

The role of the CHI is inspection of NHS facilities, structures and processes.[16] It will operate independently of the NHS trusts and health authorities, and will consist of multidisciplinary teams including doctors and nurses. The BMA welcomed the initiative,[17] which for the first time brings the NHS under external scrutiny.

All of the above policies emphasise 'performance' and 'self-regulation'. Clinical governance places on doctors the statutory duty for increased accountability both for the provision of health and for efficiency. Doctors in the UK have never been closely regulated, with the GMC taking about a century and a half to set up a system to deal with poorly performing doctors.[18]

The changes in 1999 brought in a fundamental change in that respect, since for the first time 'good performance' includes not only the standards set by the GMC, but also those laid down by external bodies such as NICE and CHI. Doctors now face the prospect of compulsory revalidation and audit of their clinical activity by their PCG/PCT.[19]

It has been pointed out that such changes embody 'a great deal of logic' – revalidation makes sense given that doctors need to continually update their knowledge, skills and attitudes.[20] Nevertheless, a large number of articles published in the *British Medical Journal* (*BMJ*) since 1998 are devoted to the potential conflict of interests between the PCG's responsibility for clinical governance and the GP's independent contractor status. The issues include the risk of compromising clinical freedoms (especially freedom to prescribe because of financial pressures), the motivation of GPs if they are over-regulated, and public respect for the medical profession.[21]

Alongside policy initiatives that appear to emphasise regulation there are influences which emphasise the role of education in bringing about change. For example, in 1998 the *Chief Medical Officer's Review of Continuing Professional Development* was undertaken and published with the aim of producing 'improved patient care underpinned by evidence and a valued process of development.'[22] The 'Learning as a Lever to Deliver Change' project is operating within this context, attempting to establish the GP tutors' educational role as critical to the ambitious change agenda, which 'is not merely about managing people, but about educating, sharing a corporate vision, disseminating knowledge and understanding in a culturally sensitive way. It will require expert change management, creating the right philosophy and environment for professionals and practices to flourish.'[23]

With this in mind, the next section examines in more detail the role of the GP tutor as a key agent of change.

The perceptions of GP tutors

The empirical part of the evaluation consisted of interviews with six GP tutors who were asked to describe their activities and experiences, and to give their views about their role. The interview transcripts were analysed in order to ascertain the main points, which were then sent back to the GP tutors for comment. This has ensured a more accurate account of their perceptions. The value of exploring the GP tutors' perceptions and experience lies in understanding what (for what can be regarded as a group of key change agents) are the main issues and workable models of facilitating education.

The next section examines the GP tutors' perceptions of the context of change – their role, activities and experience, and the evolving shape of reforms.

The context of change

There is a general perception that a 'culture change' is taking place. Perhaps as a form of shorthand, most suggested that this is marked by the establishment of PCGs (in April 1999). However, one pointed to the documents and developments discussed in the previous section as the markers of change, observing that 'all of this CPD change could have happened without them [PCGs].'

None the less, there was agreement that healthcare professionals, including general practitioners, were being required to work differently in the following ways:

- aligning individual personal and professional development to local (PCG and HA) and national (NHS) interests and priorities, and demonstrating that this was being done
- demonstrating competent performance for revalidation
- working in multi- (or inter-) professional teams
- being accountable to a variety of interest groups
- building relationships with patients on a more equal basis.

Although some GP tutors were, to varying degrees, anxious about the final shape of reforms, there was general acceptance of the need for such changes. The general perception is that a more rigorous approach to the continuing education of doctors will result in an improvement in health (*see* below).

The GP tutors' perception of their role

The GP tutors' initial plans focus on ways of encouraging GPs to understand and respond to the current reforms. However, their aims and practices as GP tutors are more complex and subtle than this might suggest. They see themselves as educational facilitators and peers who can help colleague healthcare professionals 'survive and thrive' within these changes. They construe the way in which they set about this in a variety of ways, including the following:

- encouraging people to take responsibility for their own learning
- increasing GPs' interest and enjoyment in their work
- improving courses
- providing a forum for airing views
- helping those who are struggling in a positive way
- stimulating ideas
- nurturing and leading
- encouraging reflective practice
- helping people to make connections between individual aspirations, everyday work in the practice and the outside context of the PCG and national priorities
- helping people to appreciate and use the educational resource that already exists within their primary healthcare teams.

Thus educational expertise is understood as knowledge of processes of change and as the ability to encourage self-education. The next section will examine how this is put into practice.

Activities

It is important to emphasise that GP tutors conduct their activities under considerable time constraints. They have one or two sessions a week (that is, two to four hours), and they work with PCGs consisting of between 6 and 30 practices of different sizes.

In general, the GP tutors consider that CPD needs to balance individual, practice, PCG and national interests. This definition of CPD guides their choice of activities. Individual GP tutors have different emphases because they work in different geographical areas of variable size and nature with different features (e.g. number of single-handed practices) and different histories and traditions of educational activities, and GP tutors themselves have different areas of expertise and interest.

Nevertheless, the trend is the same for all. The 'traditional' GP tutor work of organising courses in different centres continues, and the aim is to encourage GPs to choose topics that are relevant to PCG and national priorities. However, the idea is to change the 'credit-accumulation' view of education that is encouraged by the PGEA system, to move away from traditional lecture delivery, and to work towards more engaging forms of education that are in-practice, work-based and interprofessional.

In addition to courses and events held in centres in the evenings or at lunchtime, GP tutors have undertaken the following activities:

- visiting practices (sometimes talking one-to-one and sometimes to groups) in order to explain current reforms
- use of questionnaires to establish educational needs
- meetings with clinical governance leads and others
- being used as a resource to help established groups
- written a guide to the new arrangements for GP education and PGEA
- devising a model and example for personal development plans (PDPs) and a model for practice professional development plans (PPDPs)
- co-ordinating activity (e.g. newsletter)
- multiprofessional CPD group
- helping non-principals with their PDPs.

Experience of their role

GP tutors are enthusiasts, and some of them have long experience of educational work. They believe in what they are promoting and enjoy working with colleagues, many of whom appear to be grateful to them for their help and attention. There are new challenges for which new skills are required (e.g. working within different disciplines, supporting CPD with primary healthcare teams, and conducting appraisals).

There are differences in the extent to which they accept current changes. For those who are more hostile to change, the major problem is the threat to professional autonomy (*see* below), and also the fact that personal professional development is considered to be the central focus of CPD. Others acknowledge an historical and cultural barrier in the profession to making explicit links between the individual and state priorities, but at the same time they consider that there are benefits. There is a general perception that there is too little time, support and resources to fulfil the role.[24]

The evolving shape of reforms

There is a strong sense that matters are not yet settled. The major outstanding issue in this respect is the extent to which the approach to improving the service will be facilitative or regulatory.

On the whole, GP tutors acknowledge that there is a need for change in the system,[25] and they are not resistant to the idea of greater accountability and to improvement based on evidence. However, they are opposed to the policies and practices of a whole system being driven by a concern about 'poor performance'. Some GP tutors sense that government is treating the profession as untrustworthy;[26] and most of them are not confident that, despite being involved in good practice, they will have any influence on the final shape of the reforms. They also perceive a shift from encouragement to demands. Two examples illustrate this lack of clarity and will be discussed here.

Personal development plans (PDPs)

The requirement for PDPs (and for PPDPs), originally required by April 2000,[27] is perceived as a key factor in motivating general practitioners to learn and develop skills. However, the nature and purpose of the PDP is critical. There are two main ways of viewing these:

- as a vehicle for ensuring that work is done to a high standard, and for making connections between personal development and local and national health priorities
- as an instrument of surveillance, monitoring performance and identifying 'poorly performing' doctors.

In this respect a tension is perceived between the GP tutor's role of facilitating the development of a meaningful PDP and the clinical governance lead's role of 'signing off' PDPs.[28] It is speculated that a PDP is not signed off because of 'poor performance' or because it is not in line with PCG, HA and NHS priorities.

It is still uncertain who will undertake appraisal, and the nature of the relationship of PDPs to the identification of 'poor performance' is also still unclear, although at present it is viewed as relatively informal. One GP tutor suggested two possible models:[29]

> one is that there should be some form of appraisal underpinning the PDP and its development. The ideal would be a one-to-one with a GP tutor, a sort of educational overview and dialogue ('professional conversation' model). However, time commitments mean in reality we cannot do a one-to-one with all, so self-appraisal methods, using tools that we have helped to devise, or group appraisals within practices will be used, with some one-to-ones ... However, revalidation includes some form of appraisal and the feeling is that this will be an altogether different affair with different motivators and aims – a less friendly, more judgemental interview – really a performance review.

The questions raised are whether there will be two parallel schemes, and whether it is at all possible to reconcile the differing aims of appraisal. Much will depend on the final form that revalidation takes. At the same time, it is likely that doctors will dispute what is best for patients, despite the setting of national standards.

The clinical governance lead

The GP tutors hope that GP tutor and clinical governance lead roles will be complementary (one GP tutor is also a clinical governance lead). Both are aimed at improvement of quality through some type of educational endeavour. GP tutors view themselves as working in co-operation with clinical governance leads. However, there was anxiety that the role of the latter will involve 'stick', and that objectives will start to become incompatible.

To conclude this section, GP tutors point out that GPs are already demoralised by having to respond to organisational change that they do not always believe is desirable. They predict that if GPs feel that they are being dictated to, they will begin to 'cheat the system' (however, GP tutors do not see their role as helping colleagues to do this). Reactions will be negative if changes are perceived as too fast and/or under-resourced. Authentic improvement must rely on self-direction and professional values. From the GP tutors' point of view, over-prescriptive, threatening, over-burdensome or complicated systems of accountability and quality improvement will militate against genuine and desirable change.

Discussion

The conventional method of evaluation is to return to aims and objectives and to use evidence to judge the extent to which they have been achieved. However, it is often the case that during the course of a project its objectives change. In the case of the 'Learning as a Lever to Deliver Change' project, this process has been sharper than usual because it has been conducted during a period of rapid and (it may be argued) turbulent change for GPs. As the pressure to establish systems of monitoring and accountability appears to increase, a major issue has been the extent to which GP tutors, as professionals and educators, can be viewed as (one group of) mediators between state regulation and professional self-regulation.

Accountability, regulation and autonomy

A strong theme emerging from this evaluation is that medical professionals perceive unresolved tensions. The tension one is between government control and professional autonomy. In connection with this there is the tension in systems of accountability and regulation between punitive or enabling functions. More specifically, there is the tension between improvement of service through a focus on audit and standards on the one hand, and through attention to the quality of relationships between a range of individuals, groups and agencies on the other.

The need for regulation and accountability is accepted, but the form that it will take is still evolving, and the profession has been wary in response to the dictatorial tone of the *Supporting Doctors, Protecting Patients* document written by the Chief Medical Officer earlier this year. It has been suggested in this document that the shift from self-regulation to self-regulation under external scrutiny is inevitable,[30] but that there are grounds for believing that the shape of self-regulation can be and is being negotiated by members of the profession. These grounds are found both in precedents and in the efforts currently being undertaken by, for example, professional bodies and GP tutors.

Bearing in mind that most of the group of GP tutors who took part in the evaluation study were not optimistic about their ability to influence change, there may be something to learn from the experience of teachers in the last 20 years. There is a good deal of research about teachers' responses to increased regulation and managerial demands. While much of it identifies 'deprofessionalisation' and demoralisation,[31] this view is rarely unequivocal. Teachers cope in a variety of ways that include resistance and 'reprofessionalisation' or 're-skilling'. It appears that state policy is rarely passed down as intended, but rather it is interpreted in different contexts and at different levels.[32] There is a limit to the state's capacity to manage.[33] There are then 'spaces' in which good practice (defined as such by the profession) could be established.

It has been pointed out that the medical profession has not strongly resisted the current proposals for regulation, and it has been suggested that compliance has followed from media and public responses to accounts of malpractice.[34] This may in turn result in further problems. Dr Ian Bogle, the BMA chair, warned that 'procedures designed for a minority of doctors could be seen as threatening all doctors, further lowering morale'.[35]

However, Buetow and Roland argue that 'if successful, [clinical governance] will define a new type of professional for the next century. Failure by the professions to seize the opportunity is likely to result in [the] increasingly detailed external … and tight managerial control found in some other countries'.[36]

Opportunities are already being negotiated. For example, the RCGP responded quickly to *Supporting Doctors, Protecting Patients*,[37] and followed this with a discussion document describing a framework of accountability, including regulation of the profession, and a model for the future. This was written with the following specific aim: 'to develop an understanding of how we wish to influence thinking on a system of regulation that meets the needs of the profession, patients and the state.'[38] At the level of CPD for GPs in the West Midlands region, a strategy document develops a framework which builds on a long experience of supporting the CPD of GPs, and which includes clearly defined functions and roles for the GP tutor.[39] This is the context in which the GP tutors work, and which forms the backdrop to any discussion about their future role and direction.

The future of the GP tutor role

The evaluation set out to explore the significance of the GP tutor role. However, this aim has been overtaken by clear statements that they will be key to successful change. Since the evaluation project began, the role of the GP tutor has been promoted in both regional and national documents. *The West Midlands Regional Strategy* (February 2000)[40] proposes a 'two-tier' model consisting of GP tutor support at PCG[41] and health authority levels, and includes job descriptions. The Royal College of General Practitioners (RCGP) (April 2000)[42] recommends a 'new network of education tutors'. The region envisages two GP tutor sessions per 100 000 patients, while the RCGP recommends ten sessions for every 50 general practitioners.[43]

The role of the GP as educator is already well established in the area of vocational training. It is now seems that a role reconfigured to emphasise working with practices, interdisciplinary teams and individuals has been accepted for the future.

This evaluation suggests that the confidence is well placed, perhaps because GP tutors come to their work with a particular interest in education, they are exceptionally 'good value for money', they are committed, enthusiastic, capable and energetic, and they cover a great deal of ground in the short time that is available to them. Perhaps more importantly, they appear to be particularly well placed as 'change agents'. They can 'read' the history and traditions of the area in which they work, and adapt their activities and approaches to take into account the conditions of their particular context. They are likely to understand what will motivate the GPs with whom they are working, and this is appreciated: 'I hope that this meeting is an indication of the evolution of a supportive structure for GPs who are under increased pressures in the face of government demands and increased patient expectation'.[44] They are also well positioned to identify common issues across practices.

With regard to the future, the three managers who were interviewed[45] concurred with the GP tutors about purpose, direction and values. They envisaged GP tutors as continuing to work with individuals and practices to establish needs and plans which integrate the demands of different interest groups. They also saw GP tutors making opportunities available for meeting needs and being a focus for multidisciplinary education. Furthermore, they stressed the importance for genuine improvement of avoiding 'prescription and heavy monitoring',[46] and they regarded the GP tutors as introducing change by 'dealing with GPs in a non-confrontational, non-threatening manner.' [47]

The next section looks at representations of the GP tutor's work.

'Models' or 'principles of practice'?

A major aim of the original evaluation project was to describe and examine 'models' of working as a GP tutor and to 'determine an optimal role'. However, GP tutors' work defies models. As part of the evaluation, they were asked to provide diagrammatic representations of their work. Their responses indicated that, although certain elements might be common, the work is complex and can be conceived of in different ways. Thus it is both likely and desirable that there will be 'customised versions'[48] of the GP tutor role.

There are several reasons for this. Local conditions differ in many respects (e.g. in the comparative numbers of single-handed and group practices, the number of training practices, whether the area is largely rural or industrial). These conditions may have an impact on what can be called an area's 'readiness' for change and innovation (e.g. the degree to which there is a history of collaboration between doctors, with other healthcare professionals and with postgraduate centres of medical education). This is not straightforward. For example, GPs in neglected areas may be particularly receptive to the attentions of a PCG which is communicating with previously isolated practices,[49] while GPs in areas where there are already developing systems of improvement and quality assurance may resent requirements to work in different ways. In addition, GP tutors themselves differ in their expertise, experience and preferred ways of working.

Beyond descriptions of duties and responsibilities,[50] it may be helpful to consider GP tutors' work in terms of common 'principles of practice'. Some are already evident. For example, GP tutors aim to engage GPs in taking an interest in and being responsible for their own CPD, and to encourage them to articulate relationships between individual, practice, local and national interests. They are also working hard to gain acceptance and negotiate agreements about what needs to be done and how. One manager put it like this:

> It is very important to work with the existing mind-set because things can't be done overnight ... It is about ... doing sensible, constructive, positive things that help them keep up to date. The agenda is to get them to work together ... then, some years down the line, when there is a body of consensus about basic issues, we can begin to tackle the more difficult ones ... we are after consensus about what suits us locally. [51]

In the mean time, the Government is unlikely to cease demanding evidence that attempts at CPD are having an effect. There is a need for GP tutors and their managers to consider how to make convincing accounts of their work.

The need to review and build up an 'evidence base'

One of the original aims of the project was to demonstrate the way in which the GP tutor role results in 'improvements in care of individual patients'. This is unlikely to be possible within the timescale available. Grant and Stanton[52] have made the following point:

> *The huge range of variables which have the potential to intervene at the different stages of the CPD process illustrates the complexity, if not the impossibility, of trying to assess the influence of an educational activity on professional behaviour or practice outcomes.*

In their study of 15 GP tutors, Singleton *et al.*[53] insist that 'any critical assessment [of GP tutors' work] should be context based, and sympathetic and responsive to local conditions'. This does not amount to an argument for making no attempts to evaluate. On the contrary, it is imperative that GP tutors pursue their own evidence base for what they are doing. This is particularly so both because there is no educational right method, and because there is substantial evidence that effective CPD involves attention to processes and culture.[54]

GP tutors need systems of self-review and evaluation that address the complexity and qualitative nature of their educational work, and that are not over-burdensome, but which nevertheless can be presented as evidence. It appears that, at present, in general GP tutors' time and commitment are devoted to planning and doing, and the review of effects is comparatively neglected.[55]

Evaluation should not be confused with time-consuming efforts to collect a large amount of quantifiable measures. In fact, there are dangers:[56]

> *In complex fields of practice, there is a risk that assessment highlights the readily measurable, over-emphasising detail rather than promoting essential aspects of competence. In this way, practice is trivialised through assessment that fails to support professional development.*

Professionals can argue about what counts as evidence in their field of practice, and conclusions always involve interpretation, which incorporates professional judgement.[57] Critical evaluation that builds up knowledge about what works and what does not in different contexts could provide a further 'principle of practice'.

Conclusion

Medical practice in contemporary conditions requires reflective, self-educating professionals who are capable of delivering effective healthcare both to individual patients and to populations, and of working within a constantly changing NHS and society. It is no straightforward matter to achieve this, and individual practitioners are likely to need support. The GP tutor can provide this support.

This project and its evaluation have taken place on shifting ground. A plethora of documents superseding each other charts the evolution of reforms which centre on the notion of 'revalidation'.[58] Many of the policy initiatives and messages are contradictory, or at least have a dual potential. As suggested in *The West Midlands Regional CPD Strategy*,[59] the key to reconciliation appears to lie in grasping and making use of the overlapping relationship between professional self-regulation and lifelong learning.

The GP tutors, along with many other players, can play a crucial role in this task and possibly become influential mediators of policy. The need for change is broadly accepted. Time and resources are needed to develop systems and practices that improve practice and are workable within different contexts and constraints. It has been suggested that it is important to attempt to negotiate a way of working and of accounting for work which reflects what medical practice really is. It has been argued that general practice involves a great deal of uncertainty, but that it is the dilemmas that this raises which engage GP energy and enthusiasm.[60] If this is true, it is important not to misrepresent the nature of GP work to the public.

The degree and nature of control over the profession have not been clarified. One GP tutor has remarked that 'It is interesting where we will be in time – still a peer and advocate or part of the system passing judgement at the same time as it hands out remedies?'[61] This will depend on the form that 'revalidation' takes. If it is based on personal portfolios and local validation, much good work could continue and be developed.

The enthusiasm and entrepreneurial skills of individual GP tutors urgently require a national framework that sets out the service expectations of GP tutors, and their funding and responsibilities within clinical governance, revalidation and lifelong learning.

Acknowledgements

The authors wish to thank all of the doctors and managers who gave up their time to contribute to the study.

References

1   Fisher MJY (1999) *Funding Submission*. University of Keele Centre for Primary Care with the Director of GP Education West Midlands Region, 18 June.

2   Five days undertaken by the Education Department, University of Keele.

3   The original intention was to focus the evaluation on group discussion with GP tutors, but convening six GPs at the same time proved impracticable.

4   Fisher MJY (1999) *Funding Submission*. University of Keele Centre for Primary Care with the Director of GP Education West Midlands Region, 18 June.

5   In relation to GPs, the Shipman case has been particularly potent.

6   Johnson T (1984) Professionalism: occupation or ideology? In: S Goodlad (ed.) *Education for the Professions: Quis custodiet ...?* Society for Research into Higher Education and NFER-Nelson, Windsor.

7   These questions were raised in relation to states and welfare systems in general, not the UK only.

8   Bottery M (1998) *Professionals and Policy*. Cassell, London. Also Clarke J and Newman J (1997) *The Managerial State*. Sage, London.

9   ibid.

10 For example, Ozga J (1995) Deskilling a profession: professionalism, deprofessionalisation and the new managerialism. In: H Busher and R Sarah (eds) *Managing Teachers as Professionals in Schools*. Kogan Page, London. Freidson E (1983) The theory of professions: state of the art. In: R Dingwall and P Lewis (eds) *The Sociology of the Professions: Lawyers, Doctors and Others*. Macmillan, London. Fournier V (undated), *Boundary work and the (un-)making of the professions*. Centre for Social Theory and Technology, Keele University, Keele.

11 For detailed comparisons of the three sectors, see Bottery M (1998) *Professionals and Policy*. Cassell, London.

12 Information given in feedback on draft report (F[3], 8/20).

13 For a detailed description of the White Paper and its implications for primary care practice, see Baker M (1998) *Making Sense of the New NHS White Paper*. Radcliffe Medical Press, Oxford.

14 McColl A, Roderick P, Gabbay J, Smith H and Moore M (1998) Performance indicators for primary care groups: an evidence-based approach. *BMJ.* **317**: 1354–60.

15   At present these have been developed for coronary heart disease and mental health.

16   It can be seen as the equivalent of the Office for Standards in Education (OFSTED) for schools.

17   Ashraf H (1999) Watchdog set up to monitor UK health care. *Lancet.* **354**: 1623.

18   Smith R (1998) Regulation of doctors and the Bristol inquiry. *BMJ.* **317**: 1539.

19   Richards P (1998) Professional self-respect: rights and responsibilities in the new NHS. *BMJ.* **317**: 1146. Smith R (1998) Regulation of doctors and the Bristol inquiry. *BMJ.* **317**: 1539.

20   This view was expressed by a Director of Health Policy and Public Health (8/2000), but was also held by all of the GP tutors who were interviewed.

21   Beecham L (1999) Government sets out vision for clinical governance. *BMJ.* **318**: 832; Warden J (1999) GMC advises trusts on governance. *BMJ.* **318**: 1230.

22   Chief Medical Officer (1998) *Review of CPD.* Department of Health, London, p.18.

23   Fisher MJY (1999) *Funding Submission.* University of Keele Centre for Primary Care with the Director of GP Education West Midlands Region, 18 June.

24   Corroborated by the Royal College of General Practitioners (April 2000, *see* note 7), who describe the network of GP tutors as of 'high quality', but 'under-resourced and inadequate' (p.30).

25   Not only because of 'problems', but because the social, economic and political world in which doctors work is changing.

26   For some, the consultation paper *Supporting Doctors, Protecting Patients*, written by the Chief Medical Officer on how to deal with poor clinical performance, is an indicator of lack of trust.

27   Department of Health (1998) *A First Class Service: Quality in the New NHS.* Department of Health, London.

28   The *Regional Strategy* (West Midlands Postgraduate General Practice Education Unit, February 2000) distinguishes between a PDP and an 'educational portfolio' (p.13).

29   In correspondence received on 25 May 2000.

30   Indeed, Harrison and Ahmad argue that medical autonomy has been declining over the last 25 years.

31   For example, Goodson I and Hargreaves A (1996) Teachers' professional lives: aspirations and actualities. In: A Hargreaves and I Goodson (eds) *Teachers' Professional Lives.* Falmer Press, London.

32   Bowe R and Ball SJ with Gold A (1992) *Reforming Education and Changing Schools: Case Studies in Policy Schooling.* Routledge, London.

33 Harrison S and Ahmad W (2000) Medical autonomy and the UK state 1975 to 2025. *Sociology*. **34**: 129–46.

34 ibid.

35 McIntosh K (1999) Health authorities will have powers to ... doctors in performance. *Health Serv J*.

36 Buetow SA and Roland M (1999) Clinical governance: bridging the gap between managerial and clinical approaches to quality of care. *Qual Health Care*. **8**: 184–90.

37 Royal College of General Practitioners (2000) *Response to 'Supporting Doctors, Protecting Patients'*. Royal College of General Practitioners, London.

38 Royal College of General Practitioners (2000) *The Future of Professionally Led Regulation for General Practice*. Royal College of General Practitioners, London.

39 West Midlands Postgraduate General Practice Education Unit (2000) *Continuing Professional Development in General Practice – the Regional Strategy*. WMPGPEU, Birmingham.

40 West Midlands Postgraduate General Practice Education Unit (2000) *Continuing Professional Development in General Practice – the Regional Strategy*. WMPGPEU, Birmingham.

41 Or primary care trust (PCT).

42 Royal College of General Practitioners (2000) *The Future of Professionally Led Regulation for General Practice*. Royal College of General Practitioners, London.

43 A great deal more time than this group of GP tutors have available.

44 From Dr B's report, April 2000.

45 Primary care medical adviser, a director of health policy and public health and a PCG chief executive.

46 MA: 26 June 2000.

47 CE: 12 May 2000.

48 MA: 26 June 2000.

49 CE: 12 May 2000.

50 West Midlands Postgraduate General Practice Education Unit (2000) *Continuing Professional Development in General Practice – the Regional Strategy*. WMPGPEU, Birmingham, 20–21.

51 CE: 12 May 2000.

52 Grant J and Stanton F (1999) *ASME Occasional Publication. The Effectiveness of Continuing Professional Development: A Report for the Chief Medical Officer's Review of Continuing Professional Development in Practice*. Association for the Study of Medical Education, Edinburgh.

53 Singleton A, Smith F and Hornung R (2000) Administrator, educator, entrepreneur, impresario, advisor, ringmaster, proxy-learner or fall-guy? The many

roles GP tutors play to accommodate obstacles in providing appropriate GP education. *Educ Gen Pract.* **11**: 288–96.

54   Grant and Stanton, ibid., p.27.

55   The exception was GP tutor B, who has undertaken an evaluation of her work with practices. The results have been extremely positive.

56   Grant and Stanton, ibid., p.26.

57   Frith L (1999) Evidence-based medicine and general practice. In: C Dowrick and L Frith (eds) *General Practice and Ethics: Uncertainty and Responsibility.* Routledge, London.

58   In the public imagination this is coming to mean 'doctors who don't hurt us'.

59   op. cit., p.19.

60   Dowrick C (1999) Uncertainty and responsibility. In: C Dowrick and L Frith (eds) *General Practice and Ethics: Uncertainty and Responsibility.* Routledge, London.

61   GP tutor A.

26

'Inside out or outside in?' The future of education and training for GP non-principals

Bitty Muller and Rebecca Viney

Introduction

GP non-principals are a growing group within the national primary care work-force. No longer are they a small band of locums, assistants and retainer scheme doctors. They include personal medical services (PMS), pilot schemes doctors, deputising services doctors, GP associates in remote areas, retired doctors, career-break doctors, family planning doctors, drop-in centre doctors, ships' doctors, services doctors, academics, police doctors, medical directors of health authorities and public health doctors who do sessions in general practice, and sick and suspended doctors.

Until recently, these doctors have been sidelined within the medical educational system. However, over the past five years research into GP non-principals has increased our understanding of this group of doctors.

Research findings and recommendations

In 1995, Baker and Petchey highlighted the issue of doctors who are trained as general practitioners and choose to work as non-principals.[1] This was followed by further work by Dr David Wall for the Standing Committee on Postgraduate Medical Education (SCOPME), which resulted in the report entitled *The Educational Needs of GP Non-Principals*.[2] The SCOPME report concluded with the following recommendations.

1   The mechanism for regional/deanery registers of GP non-principals should be examined by all concerned.
2   Induction to a practice needs to take place for all GP non-principals. Examples of good practice should be collected and disseminated.

3   On educational grounds, a contract and/or written statement about employment terms should be given to eligible non-principals, and should specify the time available for education within contracted hours.
4   Professional career counselling should be available, and everyone should be encouraged to avail themselves of it. A nominated person with appropriate skills who is on the Director of Postgraduate GP Education's (DPGPE) staff should be given responsibility for this.
5   GP non-principals should be included in mentoring schemes in general practice.
6   The educational needs identified by this study should be brought to the attention of those responsible for planning educational activities for GPs, including practice-based education.
7   GP non-principals should be included in initiatives to help GPs to draw up personal educational and development plans.
8   Special account should be taken of the needs of locums in managing chronic disorders, and of those who spend little time in medical work.
9   GP non-principals should be routinely notified of local educational activities in the same way as principals, and should have easy access to postgraduate centres and associated libraries.
10   All GP non-principals should be provided with written information about their eligibility for educational funding. This information needs to include contact names at the agencies concerned.
11   Mechanisms need to be devised so that GP non-principals have appropriate access to financial support to meet their educational needs.
12   GP non-principals should be given adequate time for education (study leave). This needs to be specified in contracts of employment in the case of assistants and long-term locums.
13   GP non-principals should be included on the mailing lists for important publications.

The results of this research study have now been added to by a number of other studies around the UK, which show similar trends.

Study from the South Thames West region[3]

- This was a well-qualified group of doctors, the vast majority (95%) of whom were UK trained; 70% were female, and they were more likely to have postgraduate qualifications.
- The favoured educational methods were lectures and discussion of challenging patients.
- Younger doctors were more likely to prefer working in small groups and attending interactive events.

Study from the Grampian region[4]

- In total, 87% of the doctors were female.
- The median age was 35 years.
- Longer-term career plans included part-time principal (34%), part-time non-principal (21%), part-time general practice (6%) and full-time principal (2%).
- Almost one-third (32%) of the respondents had been a principal in the past. Their reasons for being non-principals should be explored.
- The main factors that are likely to determine future career plans were family commitments (60%, of whom 53% included their husband's job/career), availability of suitable posts (30%), and financial commitments (15%).
- There was a ratio of one non-principal to every 4–7 principals.
- The estimate that there are 4000 non-principals in England is likely to be a conservative one.

Study from the Mersey deanery[5]

- Of these doctors, 73% were women.
- In total, 41% had previously been GP principals.
- In total, 48% had between one and three postgraduate qualifications.
- By far the greatest barrier to education was family workload, but the cost of courses and lack of information were also a problem.
- In total, 11% indicated that they felt the need to retrain, and a further 18% were unsure about this.

On the whole, non-principal general practitioners represent a highly qualified group of doctors who cost an estimated £1.5 billion to train. With the feminisation of the medical work-force, and the increasing tendency of younger general practitioners to choose non-principal work in their early years in practice,[6] and the trend away from settling into a practice for life, greater emphasis needs to be placed on the educational needs of this expanding group of general practitioners.

Educational initiatives in place

Many regions have now appointed specific educational advisers or tutors for non-principals. Their job can be rather overwhelming, given the large number of non-principals in each region and the difficulties of setting up a register of non-principals and then keeping it up-to-date.

The National Association of Non-Principals[7] has become a body with a national medico-political profile, and it tends to represent the interests of locums in particular. This organisation together with the Department of Health has produced a filofax-sized educational portfolio which can be used by any non-principal to record learning and educational activities in an organised way.

Self-directed learning groups are often the favoured forms of educational activity for the younger female non-principals,[3] meeting in the evening when spouses or partners are available to care for children. These groups need facilitation and leadership, and GP non-principal tutors will be hard pressed to provide this for every group. However, not all doctors find that this form of continuing medical education suits their preferred learning style, and a variety of learning and educational opportunities should be on offer for these doctors, as it is for their principal colleagues.

GP returner courses are available in three regions (West Midlands, Durham and Wessex),[8–10] and Directors of Postgraduate GP Education are making increased use of the *Red Book* regulation (paragraph 38.5 (c)) which allows a further period of registrar training for GPs who have had a substantial break from practice.

Retainer-scheme doctors have benefited from the new version of the scheme that was launched in 1999 (HSC 1999/004). Educational supervision or mentoring within practice are part of the new scheme. In the West Midlands region an annual appraisal with the local GP tutor has been instituted for retainer-scheme doctors, and two study days are provided every year free of charge. Postgraduate centres are also encouraged to allow free access to educational events for this group of doctors.

In the North Thames (East) deanery, some health authorities are including non-principals in all of the education available to principals. This includes course costs, compensation for loss of income, and a database to disseminate information and *British National Formulary* books. There is a twice-yearly newsletter for non-principals which keeps them abreast of news about revalidation, personal development plans (PDPs), clinical governance and news from the General Practitioner Committee. Personal development plans have been distributed for the last two years. Several self-directed learning groups have been funded and started, and these often consist of a mixture of non-principals and principals. GP retainer doctors have an away-day once a year with a contribution made for childcare and travel. If there are funds to spare, they have been helped with the cost of courses and books. Returners are being placed in practices flexibly, depending on their need, using the funds recently released from the *Red Book* regulations (paragraph 38.5) for retraining of principals.

The future of education and training for GP non-principals

At the UKCRA conference, participants at this workshop discussed the future for this group of doctors, taking into consideration the following key areas.

What underlying principles should guide educators in managing an educational strategy for this group of doctors?

The participants agreed that anyone who works within general practice as a doctor is a general practitioner, and that the categorisation of non-principal and principal was unhelpful. The underlying principle that should be applied is that *all* doctors who work within general practice have educational needs.

What values and beliefs underpin these principles?

In the group discussion, the following issues were raised.

- Doctors who choose to work as non-principals are of the same value to general practice as their principal colleagues, and they should not be discriminated against.
- The individual learning needs of all doctors in general practice must be considered.
- Every GP (both principal and non-principal) has a responsibility for their continuing professional development (CPD), and support for development is important.
- Equity of access and opportunity for educational activities was felt to be essential.
- Flexible careers must be accepted and accommodated within the system.
- Every region should have one tutor/GP educationalist appointed with a specific remit for non-principals until the above issues are resolved.
- The lack of a register and the lack of historical funding of non-principal GP education hamper the logistics of planning educational initiatives for this group of doctors.
- It is grossly unfair that when one chooses to work as a non-principal one loses one's NHS superannuation rights, and a medico-political solution to this anomaly should be urgently pursued.

- All of these issues could be resolved if all doctors working in primary care/ general practice were salaried.

References

1   Baker M, Williams J and Petchey R (1995) GP in principle but not in practice: a study of vocationally trained doctors not currently working as principals. *BMJ.* **310**: 1300–4.

2   Oxley J and Egan J (1998) *The Educational Needs of GP Non-Principals.* Standing Committee on Postgraduate Medical Education, London.

3   Oxenbury J (1999) Appropriate education for non-principals. In: Educating GP non-principals. *Educ Gen Pract. (Suppl.)* **10**: 345–9.

4   French F (1999) Survey of GP non-principals in Grampian region (north-east Scotland). In: Educating GP non-principals. *Educ Gen Pract. (Suppl.)* **10**: 350–2.

5   Fox J (1999) A study of non-principals in the Mersey deanery. In: Educating GP non-principals. *Educ Gen Pract. (Suppl.)* **10**: 359–60.

6   Harrison J and Van Zwanenberg T (1998) *GP Tomorrow.* Radcliffe Medical Press, Oxford.

7   National Association of Non-Principals, PO Box 188, Chichester, West Sussex PO19 2ZA. Fax 01243 536428. Website www.nanp.org.uk.

8   Muller EJ (1999) The West Midlands return to general practice course 1997–98. In: Educating GP non-principals. *Educ Gen Pract. (Suppl.)* **10**: 390–2.

9   Harrison J (1998) GP Career Start Scheme in County Durham – the implications for other schemes. In: Educating GP non-principals. *Educ Gen Pract. (Suppl.)* **9**: 141–4.

10 Dubras L (1999) Re-entry the Wessex way. In: Educating GP non-principals. *Educ Gen Pract. (Suppl.)* **10**: 375–6.

27

Testing out how PPDPs will work in practice

Ruth Chambers and Gill Wakley

Health professionals are now expected to approach their continuing professional development in a more systematic way, rather than in the *ad hoc* manner that has been usual in the past. We should be moving towards team-based learning that includes everyone, whether they are a doctor, nurse, therapist, manager or non-clinical worker. Attached nursing and therapy staff, and other independent contractors such as community pharmacists, dentists and optometrists, should be drawn into practice personal and professional development plans (PPDPs) as they evolve.[1]

Individual professional development plans (PDPs) should tie in with practice-based PPDPs. These in turn should link into those of their primary care organisation (PCO). The plans will underpin the revalidation of clinicians' professional registration or the accreditation of practices and PCGs in the future.[1]

Clinical governance should be integrated in PDPs and PPDPs if learning and strategic development are to progress in the same direction, optimising the contribution from every member of a workplace team, and minimising the additional time and resources needed to carry out quality improvements.

Personal development plans will feed into a practice personal and professional development plan that will in turn feed into the education and clinical governance programmes for the primary care organisation (PCG/PCT in England or the equivalent elsewhere in the UK).

Some GPs and other health professionals just do not know where to start. Many managers do, because they are used to a culture where annual appraisals of performance are commonplace. Some GPs have started out well with personal development plans in general practice,[2] but are now puzzling about how to make them join up into a practice personal and professional development plan, at the same time as allowing other non-GP members of the team to contribute to the practice team plan.

The method being developed from the School of Health at Staffordshire University has three fixed starting points. First, the practice team focuses the PPDP on one or two priority areas that are important for the practice and which also reflect the health needs of the patient population, and the district's and national priorities (e.g. coronary heart disease or mental healthcare) in primary care settings. Secondly, the practice team integrates clinical governance into the PPDP, using the components of clinical governance as a check-list to determine blindspots in the practice team's thinking. *See* Box 27.1.

Thirdly, it is vital to evaluate whatever new activity you undertake, whether it is a PPDP or the various pieces of work within it. Therefore, practice teams should think carefully how they will evaluate the outputs of their work, before they collect information about their baseline performance or set out their timetabled action plan.

Some practices are able to select the priorities that will shape their PPDP after minimal reflection. They may have had a recent significant event (e.g. a young man dying of a myocardial infarction on the surgery premises) and are very much aware of the district and national pressure on them to respond to the national service framework for coronary heart disease. Others oscillate about choosing priorities where several members want to follow diverse topics, and they may compromise by formulating a programme that introduces these different-priority topics at various time intervals in their PPDP over the next two years. Some practices need to gather a great deal of information first in order to map out a practice profile, while others already have information about morbidity and mortality rates to hand.

All practices are at different stages of development, with varying strengths and weaknesses. Some are crippled by a fast turnover of senior staff, while others are stable but isolated from neighbouring practices and news of health policies. Whoever is facilitating the development and application of PPDPs needs to be flexible in order to be able to accommodate the practice's character-istics and state of development. The facilitator needs a great deal of experience if they are to be credible to a hard-pressed practice team who may feel reluct-ant to devote time to the application of a PPDP through practice team learning, and who may need convincing that the benefits outweigh the disadvantages.

We have found that the clinical governance check-list of 14 components (*see* Chambers and Wakley, 2000) is the most useful tool for discussion by the practice team of 'where they are now' and 'where they want to be'. Using this tool gives a more balanced approach to identifying the learning needs of all members of the practice team, so that the viewpoint of the non-clinical staff is heard alongside the clamour for evidence-based clinical practice.

Although the PPDP should be based on a systematic assessment of the prac-tice learning needs through regular audits of important clinical conditions and organisational concerns such as access, there will be other influences on

---

Box 27.1: An example of how a practice may use the check-list of the 14 components of clinical governance to take stock of their current baseline performance and shape their practice personal and professional development plan, focusing on coronary heart disease. This is not meant to be a perfect plan, but rather an everyday example.

Establishing a learning culture: We do not have a practice protocol for post-myocardial infarction. We need to determine everyone's roles and responsibilities, and we need an update of cardiopulmonary resuscitation training for everyone. We shall hold a two-hour educational session for all of the practice which we shall facilitate ourselves. Dr T and Nurse Y will plan and lead the session, as they have both been on coronary heart disease update courses recently. We shall discuss the protocol and everyone's roles and responsibilities at that session. Two future educational sessions will look at smoking cessation and weight reduction.

Managing resources and services: Our equipment is regularly checked; this includes sphygmomanometers, defibrillator, emergency bag with relevant drugs (see audits undertaken by practice manager). We need to organise receptionist and computer clerk training for compiling disease registers.

Establishing a research and development culture: We need to investigate whether there are any gender differences in treatment/investigation. The practice manager will study our referrals for investigations, including cardiology assessments, and looking at age characteristics as well.

---

the content of the PPDP, such as the practice's aspirations, new legal requirements, fashions and others' priorities.[3,4]

The practice will need to devise a way of prioritising these needs, weighing the practice interest against practice team members' personal interests where these conflict or a decision has to be made about allocating resources or paying for study leave or course fees.

The timetabled action plan should be specific, including aims and objectives, who does what and when, how new learning needs will be identified and fed into the current or next PPDP, how the PPDP will be resourced and how it will be evaluated. The final steps will involve disseminating the learning and checking that planned changes in practice and training have occurred and that the improved performance is sustained. Personal development plans should be rechecked against the PPDP to accommodate any new roles and responsibilities that evolve from the practice learning plan or the learning sessions. Regular annual appraisals should give individuals an opportunity to review and reset personal objectives and an educational programme that is in line with the PPDP and the individual's identified needs and aspirations.

Most of the participants in the workshop at the UKRA conference thought that we should build up to PPDPs from individuals' personal development plans, and that we should keep the contents relatively simple in order to avoid overwhelming practice teams, and to reduce their fears about the enormity of composing and implementing a PPDP. Thus the workshop concluded that there is no right or wrong way of producing and implementing a PPDP at present. We are experimenting with many different approaches. We can start with PDPs and build them up, or we can start with a PPDP and allocate agreed roles and responsibilities with associated education and training needs to the PDPs of all members of the team. All of the participants believed that multiprofessional team learning was likely to improve the coherence of the team and the consistency of care that they provide, although evidence for the establishment and application of PPDPs was still needed.

References

1   Chambers R and Wakley G (2000) *Making Clinical Governance Work for You.* Radcliffe Medical Press, Oxford.

2   French F and Valentine M (2000) An evaluation of the introduction of personal learning plans for general practitioners in Grampian Region (north-east Scotland).

3   Wakley G, Chambers R and Field S (2000) *Continuing Professional Development: Making it Happen.* Radcliffe Medical Press, Oxford.

4   Chambers R and Wall D (2000) *Teaching Made Easy: a Manual for Health Professionals.* Radcliffe Medical Press, Oxford.

28

The Wessex Way

Robin While and Margareth Attwood

The Wessex Way, published as *Professional Development – A Guide for General Practice*, attempts to explain not only what is meant by a practice professional development plan (PPDP) and a personal development plan (PDP), but also to provide the mechanism to make them happen. The manual takes the mystery out of professional development by explaining how to use the existing information to analyse strengths and weaknesses, priorities and needs, and it develops a plan that will improve working life on all levels. In doing so it may provide the key to meeting the requirements of a PPDP, PDP, clinical governance and revalidation all in one go. It takes a 'painting by numbers' approach, starting with health needs assessment, moving on to the formulation of a PPDP and then by identifying individual learning needs to the formulation of a PDP. It is a menu of opportunities, some of which may seem to be more relevant or useful than others. Each section gives some basic explanation together with an example and a blank form to be completed.

In 1998, the Chief Medical Officer, in a paper entitled *A Review of Continuing Professional Development in General Practice*, recommended that the key to professional development is the PPDP, from which individuals could go on to develop their own PDP. Logically this must start with a health needs assessment of the practice population, going on to look at the strengths and skill mix of the primary healthcare team. This is a good starting point, but the PPDP should be based not only on a health needs assessment and the plans and aspirations of the practice, but also on the evidence of what is going well and what is not going so well in the practice. Significant event auditing, PACT data, complaints and performance indicators provide the evidence to support a PPDP.

If a PPDP is the starting point, a PDP is just as important. It is recommended that an individual PDP should relate in some way to the PPDP. Each member of the primary healthcare team should offer to become a resource for the practice by taking on something from the PPDP into his or her PDP. All team members will of course have different learning needs and plans for the future. The manual has attempted to show how these needs might be identified, and it discusses various methods of meeting these needs. There is also a reminder of the importance of certain generic skills, knowledge and attitudes, such as consultation skills, resuscitation, medical ethics and 'looking after yourself', which are so important for everyone who works in primary care. Primary healthcare teams can use this manual as a 'hands-on' practical guide to meeting the requirements of continuing professional development, clinical governance and professional revalidation. This will provide a model to replace PGEA and fit in with the development of primary care groups and the introduction of clinical governance. It is not an exhaustive list of what can and cannot be done, but rather a framework into which one can dovetail one's own ideas.

The authors feel that the book will help to minimise the stress that GPs face in changing the profession's approach to improving quality in practice.

29

Development or monitoring?
The case of PPDPs

Anne McKee

What are personal and professional development plans? What is their function? Why are GPs being encouraged to use them for their own and their practice's development? How are those who engage with PPDPs experiencing the process? What, if anything, is being achieved?

These were some of the questions we asked at the beginning of our pilot evaluation of PPDPs in Cambridge and North-West Anglia during 1999–2000. They proved to be politically contentious questions, bringing the evaluation into the controversial interface of policy and practice. Here education is regarded either as a means of ensuring compliance with policy or as an enlightening process which enables professionals to make judgements about practice in the contexts in which they operate. In the case of PPDPs, the controversy at this interface appeared to be about the function of PPDPs. Should they be used to serve national and local care priorities, bringing practices into line with external objectives and providing a means of monitoring those who were lagging behind? Or should PPDPs develop a learning culture within practices, prioritising the needs of individuals and their practice organisation, with due regard for the confidentiality and anonymity that are needed to take risks when addressing areas of significant weakness? In reporting this controversy, we wish to explore some of the tensions inherent in employing education as an assessment tool driving both standard-setting and the pursuit of professional excellence. That tension is a tug-of-war between assessment and development.

What was the impact of this tension on the evolution of PPDPs on the ground? We observed three critical influences on how PPDPs were being interpreted, implemented and developed.

1   There was widespread uncertainty about the purpose of PPDPs, which had implications for both the designs of the tool and engagement with the process. That uncertainty related to the management of the tension between policy and practice.

2   Different implementation strategies within Cambridge and North-West
    Anglia reflected different values and cultures within the NHS – one being
    a service culture and the other a business culture. Each culture represents
    a different approach to realising change, and appears to foster different
    types of engagement with PPDPs.
3   Expectations about what could be achieved through PPDPs were high,
    but some participating practices reported that there were few resources
    to engage with the process and respond to identified needs.

The evaluation was examining the very early stages of the evolution of PPDPs
in the Cambridgeshire and North-West Anglia region. Although it is possible
to comment on the potential of PPDPs, the process was not mature enough for
it to be possible to report on the sustainability of the different implementation
strategies or their outcomes.

Introduction: the context in which PPDPs emerged

The Chief Medical Officer's *Review of Continuing Professional Development in
General Practice*[1] recommended practice professional development plans
(PPDPs) as a means of integrating and improving educational processes in
general practice. In response to this, the Cambridge and North-West Anglia
Consortium funded the evaluation of a pilot project on personal and practice
professional development planning. The evaluation commenced in June
1999. In this chapter we shall examine the experience of PPDP planning for
participants and those supporting their involvement in it, and we shall relate
the findings of the evaluation to some of the wider challenges facing medical
education today.

   The purpose of the evaluation was to maximise what might be learned
from the project in order to inform the future development of PPDPs. It was a
deceptively simple brief.

   PPDP planning was new. It was also evolving in a changing policy context,
and this was to reshape its aims and influence how those aims were interpreted by a wide range of people involved with the provision and delivery of
primary care. From the beginning, the evaluation was to encounter different
interpretations of the intentions underpinning PPDPs. These were signalled
by the changing name of the initiative. Although the proposal of the pilot
project referred to personal and practice professional development plans, the
Chief Medical Officer had referred to practice professional development plans.
The two resource centres whose task was to facilitate its implementation in
practices adopted the Chief Medical Officer's term. The change in name can

be viewed as a metaphor for the chameleon tendency of the initiative to accommodate itself to the priorities of policy-makers, professionals, managers and practitioners. Having acknowledged this change in name, we used the term practice and professional development plans (PPDPs).

At a local level, it was the task of resource centres to facilitate the PPDP process within practices. We examined how different values and philosophies within the resource centres heavily influenced what PPDP became 'on the ground' as it was introduced into the pilot practices.

The two resource centres seemed to characterise two cultures within the NHS. One is a service culture, placing emphasis on the importance of engaging with the everyday problems of practitioners and addressing those problems in the light of current professional values and concerns. The other is the newer business culture, which starts with contemporary professional concerns and with values formed at national and regional level, and examines current practice in relation to them.

The evaluation

The evaluation brief necessitated an investigative method that was capable of examining how an embryonic innovation was being understood and developed. That need suggested a qualitative approach capable of documenting what was happening, why, with what effect, and how people understood and interpreted this. Ethnographic case study was chosen as the most appropriate methodology because of its ability to explore intentions, practice and understandings within the case. This methodology has been developed and extensively trialled within educational research,[2–4] and its value in researching health-care education and policy is being increasingly realised.[5,6]

The key evaluation questions were as follows.

- What are PPDPs?
- Why are PPDPs being implemented now?
- Who is involved with or responsible for PPDPs?
- How do these stakeholders understand and interpret PPDP planning?
- What tensions and similarities are implied in stakeholder views?
- What facilitation do the resource centres offer the practices?
- How do practices experience and value that facilitation?
- How do practices go about planning their PPDPs? What goes well and why? What difficulties are experienced and why?
- How are the tensions and overlaps between the developmental needs of individual practitioners, their practices and the needs of primary care groups (PCGs) and health authorities (HAs) being managed?

The main methods employed in the research were analysis of relevant documents, interviews and observations. Consistent with a realist ethnographic methodology, the validity of the data was established through the triangulation and negotiation of accounts with participants.[2,6] The main analytical tool consisted of establishing the grounded theories of the case. A meta-analysis of these theories was conducted.[7,8]

The policy context

The purpose of PPDPs is embedded in the policy context in which they evolved. This context was rapidly changing, and different stakeholders brought their own priorities and concerns to PPDPs. The apparent ability of the PPDPs to accommodate these multiple priorities appeared to be a solution to many different problems.

What was that policy context and how did it influence PPDPs? In *A Review of Continuing Professional Development in General Practice*, PPDP emerged with an educational emphasis on personal and practice development. Here the main purpose of PPPD was to identify the training needs of individuals and the practices in which they worked. The professionally led character of PPDP and its peer review was emphasised. This educational and professionally driven view of PPDP came at a time when pressure to set standards for practice and to actively monitor those standards was mounting. *The New NHS: Modern, Dependable*[9] and *A First-Class Service*[10] provided an agenda and infrastructure to support standard-setting and its review at national and local level. National guidelines on practice would be set by the National Institute for Clinical Excellence (NICE). Primary care groups (PCGs) and primary care trusts (PCTs) provided local structures through which the delivery of care could be managed and monitored. The practice of individuals was to comply with national priorities, but it was also to be customised to meet local needs. Clinical governance was to enable local policing of care. In this climate, PPDP – with its focus on the training needs of individuals and practices – looked as if it had a role to play in the drive for standard-setting and monitoring. Yet it also promised to be a tool for self-governance. In short, PPDPs were being interpreted as a means of both facilitating professional development and assessing practice, with no clear boundary between the two processes.

As the aims of PPDP and the problems it was intended to address grew, so too did the tensions inherent in the innovation. The original educational emphasis of the Chief Medical Officer's report did not rest easily with the emerging testing implications of monitoring and self-governance. Difficulties arising from gaps between personal developmental needs and practice developmental needs had not been acknowledged, nor were there any suggestions about how to approach potential differences between practice priorities and local or national priorities. What type of process were practices piloting PPDP being invited into? Was it to be self-directed learning? Was it to be practice-directed learning? Was it to be a process of standard-setting? Could it be all of these things? What would PPDPs look like in practice and what might they achieve?

PPDPs in practice

Two resource centres (which we shall anonymise as Steeple and Sproughton) recruited practices to take part in a one-year pilot of PPDPs. The selection sampled differences in the contexts of care, the size of practices and the experience of PCGs in these areas.

Steeple: the service culture

In Steeple, the four participating practices engaged with facilitators in constructing an understanding of the purpose of PPDPs and how to begin identifying individual and practice needs. Two sets of questionnaires, one focusing on individual training needs and the other focusing on the needs of professional groups within the team, were trialled and distributed among pilot practices. The implementation strategy in Steeple had four critical characteristics:

- the unfamiliar language of clinical governance was explained
- the demands of clinical governance were related to practice activities
- confidentiality of the PPDP process was guaranteed and safeguarded
- the autonomy of practices in engaging with PPDPs and disclosing outcomes was established.

As a result of this implementation strategy, pilot practices quickly understood what PPDPs might do for them and how to engage in the process. Information about needs assessment and developmental activity remained within individual practices, creating conditions which maximised confidentiality and placed the power of disclosure in the hands of practitioners. For practices in Steeple, PPDP became an educational process driven by individuals focused on their practical problems and professional aspirations. As a method for realising change, this strategy started with individuals in their practices and moved out towards external agendas. It owes much to a service culture which seeks to improve care through the development of practitioners and the structures in which they operate.

Sproughton: the business culture

In Sproughton, five practices participated in the pilot. Two needs assessment questionnaires were designed by the resource centre co-ordinator. These essentially asked the same questions, one focusing on individuals and the other on the practice. The language of the questionnaires was that of clinical governance. The resource centre co-ordinator had intended the questionnaires to be something of a test of what individuals knew about clinical governance and whether they understood their practice organisation in clinical govern-ance terms. The completion of the questionnaires was not facilitated, leaving participants to struggle on their own. Essentially, PPDPs were seen as a means of introducing practices to and preparing them for compliance with the demands of clinical governance. The Sproughton implementation strategy had four critical characteristics:

- the unfamiliar language of clinical governance was used but not explained
- clinical governance criteria framed needs assessment
- both the resource centre and practices analysed questionnaires and the results were compared[11]
- facilitation was directed at compliance with the demands of clinical governance.

Most practices did not understand the questionnaires and were uncertain how to engage with the process. Confusion about who should analyse the questionnaires and lead on the needs analysis caused a lengthy period of in-activity within the practices. The resource centre co-ordinator and facilitators met with practices to clarify both the language of clinical governance and the intended process. By this time most of the practices felt frustrated with and hostile towards PPDPs, and their participation became instrumental. If PPDPs were about meeting an external clinical governance agenda, they targeted those areas that would have resource benefits for their practices, such as information technology (IT) improvement. This implementation strategy owes much to the more recent business tradition within the NHS which seeks to ensure that practice performance complies with externally agreed criteria.

Stakeholder perspectives

Both Steeple and Sproughton resource centres had offered PPDPs as a means of preparing for clinical governance. Practices wanted clarity about the relation-ship between PPDPs and clinical governance. In particular, they wanted to know what could happen if they consistently identified needs which suggested that their performance was below standard. On interviewing representatives of the health authority (HA) and primary care groups (PCGs) we were unable to obtain a clear answer to that question. One respondent simply suggested that it would depend on the individual circumstances of each case. However, although the specifics of individual instances are unique, the question for practices was what sort of things could happen to those whose practice was unsatisfactory. This was a question about how clinical governance would respond to cases of repeated concern. Perhaps there was no clear answer to this question because none had yet been formulated.

The HA and PCGs we spoke to emphasised the importance of supporting primary care professionals in ways that raise the standards of delivery of care. They combine a developmental role with a policing role. It was not clear to us what the boundaries between those roles were, or how those boundaries were managed.

Findings

As noted earlier, in evaluating the pilot of PPDP we are examining this innovation in the early stages of its development. Reliable outcome measures are not yet apparent, and the potential of implementation strategies is not fully realised. With these caveats, we can identify issues which impact on the future development of PPDPs and some lessons to be learned from how it is operating on the ground. These include the following:

- the impact of implementation strategies on how practices understood and experienced PPDP
- how practices engaged with PPDP and what they did
- how the two implementation strategies positioned PPDP in relation to the external professional agenda
- resource issues.

The impact of implementation strategies

In Steeple the implementation strategy sought to make both PPDPs and clinical governance understandable and to relate them to current practice. This enabled participants to engage quickly with the innovation, shaping it to meet the emerging needs of individuals and professional groups. The underpinning intention of this strategy was to enable practices to drive their own development, first taking account of the context in which they operated and then considering the demands of an external agenda reflected in clinical governance.

In Sproughton the implementation strategy started by testing the understanding of individuals about clinical governance and the practice in which
they worked. Confused about what PPDPs were and how to engage with them,
practices became frustrated and at times hostile towards the innovation.
Resource centre intervention to clarify understanding and facilitate the PPDP
process enabled participation. The underpinning intention of this strategy
was to start with the external agenda of clinical governance and encourage
practices to use that to drive development.

What practices did

The earlier engagement of Steeple practices with PPDPs meant that they
undertook a wider range of developmental activities than did Sproughton
practices. They were also more persuaded of the utility of the innovation.
Practices in both areas initially held 'whole' practice meetings to start the PPDP
process. After that, the Steeple practices tended to meet in uniprofessional
groups, moving from an individual perspective to that of their professional
group. In contrast, Sproughton practices tended to continue meeting as a whole
practice group before meeting in multiprofessional groups. This appeared to
allow a process of mapping an external agenda down through the practice. Some
staff, particularly receptionists, felt that they could not make a contribution
to these discussions. The Sproughton practices were more likely to perceive
the PPDP process as GP led and not of equal benefit to all the practice staff.
Issues about who led the process – and for whose benefit – were still being
voiced as the evaluation came to an end.

The range of developmental activities in which practices from Steeple and
Sproughton engaged fell into three broad classifications, namely administrative
and organisational, management and clinical.

Box 29.1:   The service approach – typical PPDP activity in Steeple

Administrative	Updating protocols
and organisational	Housekeeping duties (e.g. fire drills and alarms)
	Administrative training (e.g. telephone skills)
	IT training
	Interpersonal training (e.g. dealing with aggressive patients)
	Administrative task allocation
	Messaging patient queries
	Disseminating information (e.g. newsletters)
	Uniprofessional meetings
	Multiprofessional meetings
	Whole practice meetings

continued opposite

Management	Practice view
	Identifying professional leads
	Appraisals
Clinical	Updating nursing protocols (e.g. wound treatment)
	Reviewing GP protocols (e.g. diabetes)
	Cascaded training for nurses (e.g. leg ulcers)
	Delegation of clinical care (e.g. asthma)
	Invited expert input (e.g. mental health)

Box 29.2:   The business approach – typical PPDP activity in Sproughton

Administrative and organisational	Review of selected procedures through clinical governance (e.g. recording patient queries about treatment)
	IT training
	Central memo book
	Multiprofessional meetings
	Whole practice meetings
	Dissemination of information (e.g. newsletters)
Management	Clinical governance view of practices
Clinical	Multiprofessional discussions (e.g. diabetes)
	Doctor led and disease focused
	Approached through clinical governance

Implementation strategies, PPDPs and the external agenda

We have characterised the implementation strategy of the Steeple resource centre as reflecting a service culture, and that of Sproughton as reflecting a business culture. The former shows a preference for education as an emancipatory process enabling practitioners to make autonomous judgements in relation to the provision of care. The latter shows a preference for education as a management strategy, developing the skills and systems necessary to comply with external standards of performance. It will be interesting to see in the long term whether both foster sustainable change, and how they accommodate internal practice priorities with external visions of care.

Resource issues

Much was expected of PPDPs as a means of personal and practice development. Most practices regarded the resources offered for participation as insufficient. They argued that practices subsidised the PPDP process in the form of time, catering for meetings and payment incentives for some staff. Many practices found it difficult to find the time to engage with PPDPs. Patients tapping on the staff-room window for attention during one meeting provided a pertinent image of the conflicting demands facing those in general practice.

If practices find it necessary to subsidise the PPDP process, their perceptions about its utility and acceptability become critical.

Reflections

In the implementation of PPDPs there is much to be learned about the tensions between education and monitoring. Initially construed as a means of professional and practice development, PPDPs then acquired the aims of standard-setting. Needs analysis, a core activity of PPDP, could provide a means of illuminating poor performance. A theoretical weakness of PPDPs is the assumption that developing practice, setting standards and identifying poor performance are all the same type of activity and require the same type of tools. They are not. In practice, facilitators and users of the process showed a preference for one activity over the others, and that shaped what they did and how. If PPDPs were expected to be all things to all people, in practice they were different things depending on what they were understood to be.

There are a number of educational challenges in the current climate of monitoring standards of care. The first is to clarify the differences between the learning needs of those who lie along a continuum of poor, competent and expert practice. There are significant differences in the knowledge, skills and understandings of these groups. The second challenge is to clarify the differences between practitioners, identifying perceived educational needs and what a valid test of performance would be. These require precision assessment tools which are context-sensitive.

Identifying and supporting learning needs is an essentially educational activity. Assessing performance and policing the delivery of care is an inspectorial activity. Practitioners can reasonably expect to know which activity they are being asked to engage in. Being unclear about which process operates and when causes confusion and suspicion among practitioners on the ground.

References

1 Department of Health (1998) *A Review of Continuing Professional Development in General Practice: A Report by the Chief Medical Officer*. HMSO, London.

2 Stake R (1995) *The Art of Case Study Research*. Sage, Thousand Oaks, CA.

3 Simons H (ed.) (1980) *Towards a Science of the Singular*. Occasional Publication No.10. Centre for Applied Research in Education, University of East Anglia, Norwich.

4 Stenhouse L (1978) Case study and case records: towards a contemporary history of education. *Br Educ Res J.* **4**: 21–39.

5 Keen J and Packwood T (2000) Using case studies in health services and policy research. In: C Pope and N Mays (eds) *Qualitative Research in Health Care* (2e). BMJ Books, London, 50–8.

6 Mays N and Pope C (2000) Assessing quality in qualitative research. *BMJ.* **320**: 50–2.

7 Pope C, Ziebland S and Mays N (2000) Analysing qualitative data. *BMJ.* **320**: 114–16.

8 Meyer J (2000) Using qualitative methods in health-related action research. *BMJ.* **320**: 178–81.

9 Department of Health (1998) *The New NHS: Modern, Dependable – a National Framework for Assessing Performance*. HMSO, London.

10 Department of Health (1998) *A First-Class Service: Quality in the New NHS*. HMSO, London.

11 The individual (or personal) questionnaires were only analysed by the resource centre. However, there were no reported differences between the results of these analyses and those of the practice-based questionnaires.

30

Appraisals in general practice: the way forward

Janet Marjoram
and Bob Strachan

The importance of appraisal in professional development and general practice education is now widely accepted. Appraisal skills are at the core of continuing professional development (CPD), personal development plans (PDPs) and practice professional development plans (PPDPs). As a rule it is thought to be more beneficial for general practice if the appraisal process is driven internally. However, there are now external factors operating (e.g. the possible link to GMC revalidation).

An analysis of appraisal within training practices in Birmingham has shown that only a small number of practices operate a formal system of staff appraisal. The practice manager conducts the majority of these appraisals. Only one training practice in Birmingham was found to have a system for appraising the partners. In this instance, one doctor was nominated by his partners to undertake all of the doctors' appraisals.

Although a significant number of general practitioners have acknowledged that appraisal features strongly in the NHS plan, many factors would appear to be inhibiting the rate at which appraisal systems are introduced into general practice.

For some general practices the introduction of an appraisal system will require a change in culture. Many practices display the characteristics of a centralised power culture, with power and influence spreading out from an individual or a group. Mintzburg suggests that this type of organisation tends to be strong, proud and dynamic.[1] However, he points out that the disadvantage they have is their dependency on the ability and judgement of the central power. General practitioners must therefore take the lead with regard to appraisal.

Professor Janet Grant emphasises the difference between appraisal and performance review.[2] It is important that everyone operating the scheme is trained in appraisal interviewing, and that the aims of the appraisal scheme are communicated to all those involved, in advance of the interview situation. The appraisal interview is not an arena for disciplinary procedures. Issues relating to poor performance should be addressed independently of the appraisal process.

Time pressures

Introducing an appraisal scheme into any organisation requires sensitivity and prior consultation with those involved. The process, as with any management initiative, needs to be thought out and planned carefully. A formal discussion should take place at least once a year. Preparing for the review discussion necessitates both the appraiser and the appraisee giving consideration to areas such as current performance, development and training needs and possible future objectives. A minimum of one and a half to two hours should be allowed for the appraisal interview itself.

Although they are time-consuming, if handled well, appraisal interviews can be enormously beneficial. Appraisals are a means of improving communication, a vehicle for introducing coaching/mentoring and/or a method of supporting individuals in developing their skills and increasing their performance to their full potential. If done well, appraisals can be both motivating and inspiring.

Lack of skills

If handled badly, appraisal may result in frustration, alienation and animosity. It should never be a bureaucratic burden. Haman and Irvine reported that the techniques of appraisal and the confidence to use those skills can be achieved through a focused and well-run course.[3] The West Midlands GP Unit is now funding multidiscipline appraisal skills workshops across the 12 Birmingham primary care groups.

The success of general practice, like that of other organisations, relies to a great extent on the performance of its team. The purpose of appraisal is to review and improve on current performance whilst clarifying and discussing individuals' roles within the practice. It is an opportunity to identify and agree the learning and development needs of the appraisee (staff member or doctor), taking into account the objectives of the team and the practice as a whole. It is important that the appraiser has insight into the work of the appraisee. If a doctor is to take on the role of appraiser they will need training.

Appraisal of doctors

Appraisal may be approached in a number of different ways. The issue of who conducts the appraisal is an important factor to general practitioners. There is no rigid formula. The choice will depend on the culture of the practice and the appraisal skills and expertise of the partners and practice manager. Peer appraisal or 360-Degree appraisal may be the preferred option.

Peer appraisal

Jelley and van Zwanenberg[4] defined peer appraisal as a system whereby doctors of equal status work together, usually in pairs, using an agreed appraisal protocol that addresses issues of personal, educational and professional development. They found that peer appraisal only occurred in a small minority of practices in the northern deanery, and concluded that there was still a great deal to learn about peer appraisal.

360-Degree appraisal

360-Degree appraisal is a relatively new method which may be acceptable to general practitioners. This system differs significantly from the traditional supervisor–subordinate performance evaluation. Rather than a single appraiser, 360-Degree appraisal relies on a pool of information and perspectives gathered from a number of people who have regular contact with the appraisee. It is usual to select a minimum of five and a maximum of ten raters. Less than five would limit the perspective, and more than ten would make the system too complex and time-consuming. It is necessary to appoint a lead to ensure that the raters are appropriately selected. In the business world, customers are often included in this process, and a general practice model could include patients' comments. Once the raters have been identified, the criteria by which the individual is to be appraised should be agreed upon. The data from the raters must be analysed and summarised in readiness for the performance review.

Although 360-Degree appraisals can be extremely effective, fair and useful at their best, like any method of performance review they have potential weaknesses and disadvantages. Feedback from a multitude of sources, including one's peers, can be intimidating. The time required to select raters, fill out forms and analyse the information obtained is one of the greatest drawbacks.

Preparing for an appraisal

Many factors will affect the outcome of the appraisal. Preparation by both parties is important. Last year's objectives, possible objectives for next year and factors which may be affecting performance should all be considered prior to the interview. It may be helpful to design a prompt sheet to be completed in advance in order to facilitate this preparation. Box 30.1 illustrates the typical contents of an appraisal form.

Encouraging individuals to present evidence or examples illustrating good performance and areas where there is room for improvement enables a more objective picture to be formed.

Box 30.1:   Contents of an appraisal form

- Name and date of appraisal
- Previously agreed key work areas
- Areas of work which have been done particularly well in the last 12 months
- What has contributed to this?
- Areas of work which have been particularly enjoyed
- Areas of work which have not gone well in the last 12 months
- What has contributed to this?
- Particular strengths
- Particular weaknesses
- Skills which are not being fully used
- Training or development which would improve job performance
- Training or development which would improve career progression
- What changes would make you more effective in your work?
- Other issues

The appraisal interview

The interview and the appraiser's communication skills are critical to the success of the appraisal process. A number of doctors, particularly those involved in vocational training, should have developed good feedback skills in their role as trainers. Difficult issues should be tackled sensitively and not disregarded. MacLennan,[5] when discussing criticism, suggests that:

> *Criticism done well can increase desire to perform well, particularly if you make it clear that the behaviour is being criticised and not the person. Criticism*

done badly can make an otherwise good performer lose respect for the critic and faith in the organization.

It is essential that the appraiser understands not only what they should be aiming to achieve in their role, but also the expected standard of performance and the method by which it will be measured. Feedback on performance and guidance on how to develop and improve performance are important aspects of the appraiser's role in the interview.

The appraisal interview itself is a development tool where the appraiser skilfully guides the appraisee in assessing their own performance and taking ownership and responsibility for their performance and development. The appraiser needs to convey to the appraisee that appraisal is a purposeful part of their development. They must be aware of the abilities of the appraisee and be able to guide, assist and support the individual in making the most of their potential contribution to the primary healthcare team (PHCT).

The discussion itself should start on a positive or personal note in order to put the appraisee at ease. As with any good interview, in an appraisal situation the appraisee should be doing most of the talking, and praise should be given where it is due.

The appraisee should be encouraged to take the lead in identifying their strengths and abilities and discussing their untapped skills and potential. Areas for possible improvement and development should be discussed, and agreement on a course of action should be reached. Identification of training needs is fundamental in supporting the action.

The national agenda, including the national service frameworks (NSFs), primary care group development plan (health improvement programmes) and the needs of the population are all influencing factors when formulating a practice business plan. A business plan, together with the PDP for each member of the practice team, will give direction to the PPDP and help to identify and support the need for change.

If practices are to achieve their goals and objectives, it is essential that they identify areas for development and train individuals accordingly. Appraisal provides an opportunity to empower and motivate individuals. It is important to ensure that objectives are purposeful and challenging, linked to the practice business plan, and that the outcomes are measurable. Progress should be reviewed periodically and a review date set.

References

1   Mintzburg H (1989) *Mintzberg on Management*. The Free Press, London.

2   Grant J, Chambers E and Jackson G (eds) (1999) *The Good CPD Guide*. Reed Business Information, Sutton.

3 Haman H and Irvine S (1997) Appraisal for general practice development: an evaluation of a programme of appraisal courses held in the Northern Region in 1995/96. *Educ Gen Prac.* **9**: 44–50.

4 Jelley D and van Zwanenberg T (2000) Peer appraisal in general practice: a descriptive study in Northern Deanery. *Educ Gen Pract.* **11**: 281–7.

5 MacLennan N (1996) *Coaching and Mentoring.* Gower, London.

31

Exploring the rationale behind the use of portfolios: a report of the UKCRA workshop

John Pitts

The contents of this workshop were substantively based on a paper already published by Dr John Pitts,[1] and a presentation given by Professor Colin Coles on credentialling through the natural processes of continuing professional development at the *Credentialling Physician Specialists: A World Perspective* conference hosted by the American Board of Medical Specialties and the Royal College of Physicians and Surgeons of Canada, in Chicago, USA, 8–10 June 2000.

The aim of this workshop was to explore aspects of the use of portfolio-based learning and assessment in the field of medicine and medical education, with the objective that participants would be able to identify the strengths and weaknesses of this approach. Specific issues were sought from participants and included in the overall aims of the workshop.

The background to this work stemmed from a demand from the Joint Committee on Postgraduate Training for General Practice (JCPTGP), following a three-yearly assessment visit, for the Wessex region to establish a system of performance-based re-accreditation of its general practice trainers. In particular, this was to be targeted at the identification of 'poor' teachers. Using a panel of peer assessors recruited from around the region, videotapes on which a general practice registrar presented a 'problem' case to his or her trainer were analysed and marked against a schedule of 'effective teaching behaviours'. The reliability of judgements about individual 'components', together with an overall global judgement about performance, were studied. The reliability of individual assessors' judgements (i.e. their consistency) was moderate, but inter-rater reliability did not reach a level which could support the making of a safe summative judgement, even if the assessment of one piece of problem-based teaching could constitute a valid basis for re-accreditation.[2] Following this work, and in recognition of other considerations concerning the issue of professional competence, a 'new direction' based on portfolios was suggested.[3]

The workshop

In pairs, with plenary feedback, a short presentation and summing up afterwards, the participants were asked to address the following three questions that contribute to the rationale behind portfolios.

In terms of assessing 'mature professionals', what is the place of traditional assessment?

Discussion of the overall range of comments indicated that traditional formal examination of knowledge was believed to be less appropriate than the examination of applied knowledge and skills.

Overall, in medical education the history of assessment has moved away from knowledge testing towards applied behaviour in real or simulated situations (for a detailed review, *see* Van der Vleuten).[4] 'Mature' professionals might find the concept of resitting 'final'-type examinations rather daunting. The concept of a reflective portfolio that contains, in addition to data such as audit activity, reflection on planned learning with the understanding and reasoning that lie behind such assessment of educational needs might address some of these reservations.

What are the characteristics of professional practice?

Responses focused on two separate areas. The first was the sociological nature of being a member of a profession and its implicit contract with society. Issues of control, self-regulation, creation of knowledge and vested interests were specific examples. The other view focused on the tasks that professionals have to deal with in their day-to-day work.

As Colin Coles has stated, 'Professional practice is complex. Society asks certain people to act on its behalf to provide help and support to its members.' These people act in difficult areas in which other members of the society do not know what action to take. In fact, as Mintzberg states,[5] ' Professionalism is the exercise of discretion on behalf of another in conditions of uncertainty'. Practitioners have to decide on a course of action where it may only be possible to make a judgement on the basis of incomplete or conflicting information. Implicit in this activity is the opportunity to make mistakes. Nothing is ever completely straightforward. Uncertainty, biases, errors, differences of opinion, motives and values weaken every link that connects a patient's actual condition to the selection of a test or treatment.[6] Furthermore, in the National

Health Service, with total resource availability rationed by central government, every practitioner functions with the conscious or unconscious knowledge that everything *possible* is *not* being done for patients.[7] The exercise of discretion can therefore mean choosing not to do something for any of a range of overt or covert reasons. A major failing of performance assessments is the inability of an independent observer to see and understand something which has been chosen not to be done. Portfolio reflections represent one way in which a practitioner can address, justify, reflect on and understand such non-actions.

A further insight into the issue of professional practice may be gained by considering the two models described by Fish,[8] which probably represent two extremes of a continuum. The first is the *technical–rational model*, which assumes that professional activity is a matter of technical performance following a logical sequence as part of an efficient system. This values the technical aspects of the professional's work (measurable skills, performance and procedures that can be mastered) and logical systems and efficiency. This behavioural model assumes that professional activity consists of actions that are visible, observable and therefore amenable to measurement. The emphasis is on predetermined skills and procedures, and permanent and quantifiable propositional knowledge, and measurement strives for objectivity. Fish argues that technical accountability has to be controlled by elaborate mechanisms of assessment, inspection, appraisal and accreditation, beneath which lies the view that professionals are not to be trusted – in other words, they are not fit to exercise professional judgement. An alternative view is the *professional artistry model*, which sees professional practice as an art. It stresses understanding rather than technical skills, and it takes a holistic approach to skills and knowledge. Within a core knowledge of skills and routines, it accepts that it is not possible to know everything, and it regards open capacities and competencies that cannot be mastered as more valuable than closed ones that can be, but which are usually more trivial.[9] This model stresses investigation and reflection on practice, with the practitioner investigating and seeking insights into his or her practice. What is collected is a range of interpretations from a range of perspectives and attempts made to understand these. This model accepts the essential subjectivity of data and any interpretation that is made, and it focuses on individual insights and development. It accepts professional behaviour as self-regulating. Behind this model lies a view of professionals as deserving certain autonomy as a result of their knowledge and moral responsibility. Its view with regard to defining standards is that what is below standard is perfectly easily recognised when it is seen without the need for a complex schedule of basic competence, which in itself (unless very basic) will not be agreed upon, and if it is more detailed cannot take account of the unique practitioner in a unique practice.

More light can be shed on this area by considering the nature of professional knowledge. Eraut[10] divides professional knowledge into propositional, personal and process knowledge. While propositional knowledge resides in the public domain, and is discipline-based, personal knowledge is individually acquired by experience. Process knowledge is represented as knowing how to perform the various processes that contribute to professional action, including knowing how to access and use propositional knowledge.[10] In reality it may be impossible for an assessor to separate the various components, and any assessment of professional competence which fails to observe in some way the hidden aspects of one's expertise cannot be held to be valid. Furthermore, in practice, practitioners rely on personal experience rather than abstract concepts, and where research points to an action that does not coincide with personal experience and belief, it is the former which is regarded as more risky.[11] Schon[12] refers to many areas of professional practice as 'messy confusing problems that deny technical solution'. These may be best explored through a reflective approach, and again portfolios can provide the vehicle for recording this.

How do professionals learn?

Participants' responses immediately identified that, while there is potential for learning in any situation, the greatest source of learning was from other human beings, particularly peer professionals and patients.

As Colin Coles again has stated, 'Provided doctors can engage in collective deliberation, that is if they continuously undertake the critical reconstruction of their practice, then society can be reassured that they are in safe hands'. However, a major reason why this does not occur is because, increasingly, clinicians are not being allowed access to their 'practice community'. The main reasons why this does not occur are factors such as heavy service workloads, isolation and lack of resources.[13] A study of clinical units which trainees felt most adequately met their educational needs showed that there was a sense of community, a feeling that one was a colleague with senior clinicians, and a sense of 'criticality' – that the critical reconstruction of practice was routinely addressed.[14] Studying practice and feedback, audit, and the potential for analysing and learning from mistakes and mishaps were also identifed.

Educational theory tells us that people learn best when they reflect on their practice, identify their own strengths and weaknesses, resolve any differences between what they want to learn and what others believe they should learn, negotiate and agree learning objectives with their teachers, pursue these objectives by their own efforts, articulate their learning outcomes, agree future developments and analyse how they have learned.[15] The term 'reflective practice' underwent expansion in the 1980s with authors such as Schon. Reflective practice has been defined as the process of internally examining and exploring an issue of concern, triggered by an experience, which creates and clarifies meaning in terms of self, and which results in a changed conceptual perspective.[16] Practical experience is at the centre of professional learning,[17] and it has been suggested that educational programmes should include reflective processes based on personal experiences.[18,19] For established professionals, much continuing education is of necessity part-time. Reflective practice (and the recording of it) attenuates the problems of fragmentation, lack of cohesion and coherence, and discontinuity of contact that are characteristic of modular approaches.[20] A portfolio approach provides a clear means of capturing such processes.

In my present research, using the same panel of assessors as in the video work, their agreement when rating a series of portfolios from our prospective general practice trainers course achieved a similar (only moderate) degree of reliability, again perhaps because different areas of content have different strengths of meaning for individual assessors.[21] This issue was illustrated in this workshop by the variety of ways (all of which were valid) of interpreting the questions I posed, particularly the second question (about the characteristics of professional practice).

Conclusions and summing up

Although portfolios represent as many challenges as they may represent answers, there are reasons enough to investigate their use further. In particular, as an assessment tool, there are many challenges to address about how judgements can be made.

Doctors are not good at writing things down – doing so is not in the culture of our community of learning. This may be because of the sheer number of formal examinations we have had to survive, the difficulty of summarising messy problems, the early specialisation in secondary school away from the arts (as a result of which we work with data, not words), or the risk of commitment on paper when our actions become open to scrutiny by others.

However, portfolio-based learning has benefits that may not be derived from other forms of educational activity.[22] These include the following.

* It recognises and encourages the autonomous and reflective learning that is an integral part of professional education and development.
* It is based on the real experience of the learner, and so enables the consolidation of the connection between theory and practice.
* It allows a range of learning styles to be used according to the preferences of the learner.
* It enables assessment within a framework of transparent and declared criteria and learning objectives.
* It can accommodate evidence of learning from a range of contexts.

- It provides a process for both formative and summative assessment, based on either personally derived or externally governed learning objectives.
- It provides a model for lifelong learning and continuing professional development.

In conclusion, I hope that participants identified and considered the following points.

1 Resistance to the idea of a portfolio should be seen and understood within the prevailing culture.
2 Portfolio-based learning has the potential to explore and develop an individual's professional practice.
3 There are more purposes to assessment than regulation.
4 Any assessment method is a compromise.
5 Portfolios lean towards the professional artistry model of professional practice.
6 'Traditional' approaches to assessing portfolios are likely to prove inappropriate.

References

1 Pitts J (1999) Learning portfolios, professional practice and assessment. *Educ Gen Pract.* **10**: 423–9.

2 Pitts J, Coles C and Thomas P (1998) Exploring the introduction of a performance-based component into the certification and recertification of general practice trainers. *Educ Gen Pract.* **9**: 316–24.

3 Pitts J, Coles C and Percy D (1998) Performance-based certification and recertification of general practice trainers: a new direction. *Educ Gen Pract.* **9**: 291–8.

4 Van der Vleuten CPM (1996) The assessment of professional competence: developments, research and practical implications. *Adv Health Sci Educ.* **1**: 41–67.

5 Mintzberg H (1983) *Structure in Fives*. Prentice-Hall, New York.

6 Eddy D (1988) Variations in physician practice: the role of uncertainty. In: J Dowie and A Elstein (eds) *Professional Judgement*. Cambridge University Press, Cambridge.

7 Schwartz WB and Aaron HJ (1984) Rationing hospital care: lessons from Britain. *NEJM.* **310**: 52–6.

8 Fish D (1991) But can you prove it? Quality assurance and the reflective practitioner. *Assess Eval Higher Educ.* **16**: 22–36.

9 Passmore J (1989) *The Philosophy of Teaching*. Duckworth Press, London.

10 Eraut M (1994) *Developing Professional Knowledge and Competence*. Falmer Press, London.

11   Kozielecki J (1981) *Psychological Decision Theory.* PWN-Polish Scientific Publications, Warsaw.

12   Schon DA (1987) *Educating the Reflective Practitioner: Towards a New Design for Teaching and Learning in the Professions.* Jossey-Bass, San Francisco, CA.

13   Standing Committee on Postgraduate Medical and Dental Education (1999) *Strategy for Continuing Education and Professional Development for Hospital Doctors and Dentists.* Standing Committee on Postgraduate Medical and Dental Education, London.

14   Coles C and Mountford B (1999) *Supporting Education in a Service Environment.* Wessex Deanery for Postgraduate and Medical Education, Winchester.

15   Coles C (1994) A review of learner-centred education and its applications in primary care. *Educ Gen Pract.* **5**: 19–25.

16   Boyd EM and Fales AW (1983) Reflective learning: key to learning from experience. *J Hum Psychol.* **23**: 99–117.

17   Bines H and Watson D (1992) *Developing Professional Education.* Open University Press, Milton Keynes.

18   Brookfield SD (1986) *Understanding Adult Learning.* Open University Press, Milton Keynes.

19   Boud D and Walker D (1993) Barriers to reflection on experience. In: D Boud, R Cohen and D Walker (eds) *Using Experience for Learning.* Open University Press, Milton Keynes.

20   Morrison K (1996) Developing reflective practice in higher degree students through a learning journal. *Studies Higher Educ.* **21**: 317–32.

21   Pitts J, Coles C and Thomas P (1999) Educational portfolios in the assessment of general practice trainers: reliability of assessors. *Med Educ.* **33**: 515–20.

22   Challis M (1999) Portfolio-based learning and assessment in medical education. *Med Teacher.* **21**: 370–86.

32

CELT©: a Computerised Evaluative Learning Tool

Diane Kelly

The aim of CELT is to help general practitioners to direct their learning which is linked with the workplace. The objectives were to enable individuals to:

1   follow a structured learning process to aid learning
2   think critically about day-to-day practice in order to identify learning needs
3   be more focused in learning
4   apply learning in practice.

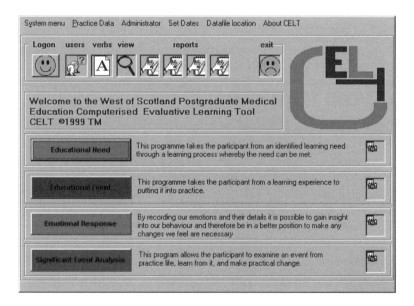

The design of CELT was based on accepted principles of adult learning theory, particularly reflective, self-directed and experiential learning. It allows an individual to develop a personalised portfolio of learning using IT. It consists of four menus, and the individual practitioner can select any combination of these. The menus are as follows.

Educational need

The user identifies a *learning need* where learning is required. The program guides the user through a process whereby the need is then met and the user is encouraged to apply the learning in practice.

Educational event

The user recalls a *learning point* where learning has already taken place, and the program enables the user to apply this in practice.

Emotional response

The user identifies a *work-related emotion* and the program guides them through a process where learning can take place and then be applied to another situation.

Significant event analysis

The user reviews a *significant event* from their working life and learns from it. The program guides the user to apply the learning to another situation.

Additional features

- The program allows the user to keep a record of their own educational activities, and allows them to track and monitor these as desired.
- The user can print reports of their learning portfolio.
- The user can email evidence of their learning direct to the Department for PGEA accreditation.
- The user can have a direct connection to the Internet for searching and access to information that is required to fulfil a learning need.
- The user can learn from day-to-day experience and develop a learning portfolio which is personally very relevant.
- The program allows the user to set their own dates for task completion and allows them to monitor their progress.
- The program enables the user to search within their own personalised database of learning activities.
- The program allows the user to track the amount of time that they spend on CELT.

CELT pilot

This was completed in August 1999 and involved 39 general practitioners, of whom 29 used CELT and 25 entered information. The evaluation consists of the following:

* pre and post questionnaires
* interviews
* analysis of entries
* awarding of sessions for PGEA.

During the four-month pilot, the 29 participants entered a total of 111 entries spread across the four menus. In 45 of these entries there was evidence of a change in practice or behaviour as a result of learning. The other outcome measure of the study was the extent to which the initial objectives had been met as ascertained from the interviews. The results will be submitted for publication, but the objectives appeared to have been met in the majority of cases. CELT was considered to be easy to use by 22 of 28 respondents.

Further developments

As a result of the analysis of the pilot, some minor modifications were made to CELT, and a CD-ROM version became available for CPD for general practitioners from April 2000.

Further development of CELT involves connection to the Web. Once this has been completed the following features will be available:

* a CELT user group where individuals using CELT can email each other (e.g. for further information where another user has a similar need)
* associate adviser feedback, where a CELT user can receive feedback on their entries prior to submission for PGEA
* in addition to each user being able to search their own database, it will also be possible for a user to search on the central database via the Web. The central database will hold details of all educational needs and objectives entered by CELT users, and individual users will be able to correspond with other users with similar educational needs
* the ability to link not only to the Internet but also to other common databases such as Medline, electronic journals, etc.

Initial steps have taken place for Phase 1 of the Web development, and this version will be piloted with a group of Scottish dentists in September 2000.

Final phase in development

Once the Web version is live, the next stage will be to develop a multi-user version of CELT. At present CELT is used by individuals for their own personal learning. The aim of the multi-user version is to have a component of CELT which links into the practice priorities and practice learning needs which can be viewed by other members of the practice team. An individual component of CELT would remain, which would only be accessed by the individual.

33

Higher professional education for general practice: a report of the UKCRA workshop

Arthur Hibble

Aims

These were as follows:

- to define higher professional education in time and educationally
- to define funding
- to define opportunities
- to define evaluations.

Method

A small group discussion was preceded by a statement of the current definitions and a short presentation by Steve Vincent, Associate Director of the Wessex deanery, of the results of a survey of the higher professional education course run in the Wessex deanery. The following is a general augmented summary of the group's discussion.

Higher professional education (HPE) in general practice

HPE can be defined both educationally and in terms of time.

The time definition describes HPE as occurring in the early years after finishing vocational training (VT), possibly in the first one to three years. This definition enables potential funders, principally the NHS in the UK, to make definite allocations and look for specific outcomes. In educational terms, HPE is the opportunity to gain additional knowledge, skills and experience that will equip the doctor for general practice within the modern NHS. This enables both the learner and the teacher to define the content, purpose and infrastructure necessary to deliver HPE. Pragmatically and politically it is likely that the profession will have to accept the time definition in order to obtain funding, and to modify the educational definition accordingly.

Discussion

A mapping study of HPE was commissioned by the NHS and undertaken jointly by the Centre for Medical Education, the Committee of General Practice Education Directors (COGPED) and the Royal College of General Practitioners (RCGP). It found that young doctors who had just completed vocational training felt poorly prepared for principalship, poorly supported educationally, and identified clear educational deficiencies in their three-year programmes.[1] During the past five years several HPE courses have been established in response to this perceived need. Many of these courses have been formally evaluated and it has been demonstrated that the needs of the newly qualified GP can be satisfied by such courses.[2]

General practice has evolved from an illness-focused service to wider disease prevention and assumed public health functions. It has changed direction from a series of small businesses responding to individual patient needs to integration into the NHS. In 1966, the Todd Report recommended five years of training for general practice at that stage. For political reasons, only three of the five years were accepted and incorporated into statute, and of these only one year in general practice was paid for.

There has often been confusion of titles and definitions with other educational events involving the words 'higher', 'education', 'training' and 'development'. At the two Cambridge conferences on HPE in general practice, in 1996 and 1998, the following definitions were agreed in an attempt to try to achieve conformity and reduce confusion.

- HPE – as above
- HPT – specific educational event courses designed to offer the learner high-level knowledge and skills applicable to general practice (e.g. certificates, diplomas and masters courses)
- HPD – the acquisition of higher-level knowledge and skills at any stage in a GP's career (e.g. masters course, writing and MD, etc.). It is often confused with HPE.

In the 1990s, several HPE courses were established in the East Anglia, Wessex, Oxford, North West and Northern deaneries. In addition, several deaneries developed short-term educational projects with health authorities to offer special opportunities of additional training posts with combinations of service delivery and supported learning. These schemes were funded by LIZEI money and the Scottish HPE posts. The aims of these various enterprises ranged from learner-centred educational need provision to facilitation of future academic or service leaders in general practice. The funding of these courses was from any of various sources, including the learners, the faculties of the RCGP, the health authorities, MADEL, LIZEI and the Scottish Medical Education Fund. Many of them were related to recruitment and retention issues in areas of particular need. Formal evaluation of these projects has demonstrated both relevance and effectiveness.[3,4]

Funding is still an issue in the UK, but there are currently possibilities of HPE being funded through the Department of Health report on acceptance of the RCGP developments in vocational training for general practice. HPT opportunities can be funded by prolonged study leave, private and public bursaries and the individual's own resources. Some primary care groups and primary care trusts are funding HPT for individuals to service specific local needs and wants.

If HPE is to be extended, then the educational establishment will need to start to define the resources required and make the necessary links with educational institutions.

There is also the issue of academic validation and acquiring credits that can be collected towards further qualifications. Some universities are now recognising vocational training and summative assessment for CATs points, which can be collected against Masters courses. There will also need to be a change in the culture of general practice service provision. Traditionally, young GPs are brought into a partnership to take a full share of the work and not to have time set aside for learning and development. There are other issues that also need to be considered, such as the need to train HPE supervisors in practice (this is a different task to vocational training). If schemes are created, we need to consider how to encourage new GPs to take part in them.

During the next few years, as various schemes and projects are started, there needs to be a central register of courses and formal evaluations to help potential participants and course organisers. It was felt that this was a job for either the RCGP or COGPED.

Training for academic general practice is a subset of HPE. At the same time as the growth of general HPE, there has been an increase in the number of posts designed to foster and develop a career in academic general practice. The Savill Report[5] recommends a two-stage progression through junior and senior levels, with the junior level corresponding to HPE. Funding for these posts would need to be incorporated into central budgets.

References

1   Grant J (1998) The higher professional education mapping exercise. In: A Hibble (ed.) *Higher Professional Education for General Practice. Report on the Second Cambridge Conference.* Postgraduate Medical and Dental Education, East Anglia Deanery.

2   White A and Severs M (1999) Training and development of doctors for general practice. *Educ Gen Pract.* **10**: 462–8.

3   Bregazzi R, Harrison J and van Zwanenberg T (2000) Mentoring new GPs. *Educ Gen Pract.* **11**: 58–64.

4   Smith LFP, Eve R and Crabtree R (2000) Higher professional education for general medical practitioners. *Br J Gen Pract.* **50**: 288–92, 293–8.

5   Academy of Medical Sciences (2000) *The Tenure-Track Clinical Scientist (The Savill Report).* Academy of Medical Sciences, London.

34

Membership by assessment of performance of the RCGP and the criteria for trainers and their practices

John Holden

Introduction

Membership by assessment of performance (MAP) offers a new route to membership of the Royal College of General Practitioners (RCGP) for experienced general practitioners who can show evidence of good-quality practice. MAP is aimed particularly at the needs of established practitioners who, for a variety of reasons, did not take the Membership Examination. The process is designed to assess the direct clinical care of patients, and the skills, organisation and professional development that underpin the quality of this care. The assessment is aimed at the individual doctor rather than at the practice, with the explicit intention that those working in general practice in roles other than as a principal and practice partner should not be disadvantaged.

The standard required for MAP is that of normal good practice as assessed by practising doctors. The scheme was developed after extensive consultation with general practitioners throughout the UK.[1] Training practices should be able to fulfil the requirements for MAP, and deaneries who have not required the MRCGP for trainers in the past are now expecting trainers to be College members or to be working towards membership.

In Box 34.1 I have compared the criteria required for MAP[2] with the attributes of trainers as doctors, and practices suitable for training, as described by the Joint Committee on Postgraduate Training for General Practice (JCPTGP).[3] The *MAP Handbook* describes in detail the evidence to be supplied, and all 36 essential criteria must be passed, together with 10 optional criteria (marked *).

Box 34.1: JCPTGP criteria for trainers and their practices, and MAP criteria

[MAP criteria are shown in italics, numbered as they appear in the Handbook]

A high standard of professional and personal values in relation to patient care
Reflected in all MAP criteria

Appropriate availability and accessibility to patients
1a *Patients who have, or consider they have, an urgent problem are able to be assessed the same working day*
1b *A system is in place to allow emergency problems to be dealt with immediately and appropriately*
1d *For routine matters, patients can see the candidate within ten of the candidate's working surgeries*

A high standard of clinical competence
5b *The candidate will be competent in emergency resuscitation*
5c *The candidate makes rational and competent decisions regarding the diagnosis of patients with a range of acute illnesses*
5d *The candidate's management of emergency admissions is competent*
5e* *The candidate ensures the provision of appropriate and competent out-of-hours care*
6a *The candidate cares for patients with chronic illness appropriately and competently*
6c* *The candidate's care of a terminally ill patient for whose clinical care he or she has had the main responsibility is appropriate*
6d* *The candidate's care of a patient with chronic debilitating illness for whose clinical care he or she has had the main responsibility is appropriate*

The ability to communicate effectively
10a *The candidate consults to a standard equivalent to that currently required for the MRCGP examination (video or simulated surgery)*
10b* *The candidate assesses patients' satisfaction with their consultations*
8a *The candidate demonstrates that there is appropriate access to him or her for urgent and routine communications*
5f* *The candidate has patient information leaflets regarding acute illness available, and is able to justify their content*

A commitment to personal, professional development as a clinician
2a *The candidate can demonstrate how he or she identified three substantial educational needs within the last five years*
2b *The candidate can demonstrate how he or she met those needs*
2c *The candidate can demonstrate that change occurred in clinical care or practice management*
2d *The candidate participates in continuing educational activities*

continued opposite

2e*   *The candidate demonstrates his or her activity in up to three of the following areas: personal research; use of investigations; skills development; evidence-based medicine. The candidate demonstrates how they chose the area to review, undertook the work and reviewed the outcome*

2f*   *The candidate demonstrates how he or she uses a reflective diary to improve patient care*

A commitment to audit and peer review

6b   *The candidate uses audits to improve his or her care of patients with chronic illness*

Partners and staff who practise a high standard of medicine, and who are committed to vocational training

8e*   *The candidate illustrates the importance of continuing professional development for the practice team, and takes part in joint learning activities*

8f*   *The candidate is involved in practice development*

An effective primary care team

8b   *The candidate identifies contact arrangements for relevant members of the PHCT, both internal and external to the practice*

8c   *The candidate communicates effectively with different members of the PHCT*

6e*   *The candidate directs patients and carers to appropriate self-help and support groups*

9f   *The candidate can ensure appropriate access for patients to the full range of nursing, professions allied to medicine, social and related services*

Involvement in quality assurance

2g*   *The candidate undertakes significant event reviews in the practice*

Well-organised practice records and registers or their computerised equivalents

7a   *The candidate makes legible and appropriate records*

7b   *The candidate knows the practice's list size and demographic features*

7c   *The candidate identifies groups of patients with important conditions*

7d   *Medical records are in chronological order and contain a summary of important events in 80% of patients*

All training practices should have methods for monitoring prescribing habits as an important part of the audit process

9a   *The candidate reviews his or her prescribing*

9b   *The candidate reviews his or her patients on repeat prescriptions*

9c   *The candidate makes appropriate use of generic prescribing*

continued overleaf

All trainers and training practices should diligently observe and teach the professional guidance contained within the GMC publications *Good Medical Practice* and *Maintaining Good Medical Practice.*

3a   *The candidate has a personal written policy to ensure confidentiality. The candidate has a working policy that demonstrates ethical handling of confidential records*

3b   *The candidate is prepared to discuss personal experience of ethical dilemmas*

3d   *The candidate does not discriminate as a clinician, a colleague and an employer*

Effective practice management
Reflected in all MAP criteria

Appropriate availability of hospital services

9d   *The candidate makes appropriate referrals to other health professionals*

9e   *The candidate critically evaluates his or her referrals to other health professionals*

A volume of practice workload which ensures a balance for the GP registrar between the gaining of clinical experience and other opportunities for learning

1c   *Routine consultations average 7.5 minutes or more contact with the doctor*

1e   *The candidate has a written policy for providing continuity of care, and can demonstrate the extent to which it is implemented*

Appropriate methods of responding to patient comments and complaints

3c   *The candidate has a complaints procedure which complies with current guidance*

Adequate medical equipment should be readily available

5a   *The candidate has access to a justifiable selection of essential in-date drugs and functional equipment*

Provision should be made for preventive care and health promotion

4a   *The candidate demonstrates how he or she undertakes health promotion/primary prevention activity in his or her day-to-day practice, taking into account local factors, in at least one area*

4b*   *The candidate is prepared to discuss up to a further three areas where he or she has carried out work to promote and improve health*

New patients should be provided with a practice leaflet describing the services provided by the practice

8d   *The candidate has an appropriate practice leaflet*

Discussion

Although the JCPTGP minimum standards for trainers and their practices have developed since 1984, and the scheme for MAP was not intended primarily as an assessment of GP trainers, trainers contributed a great deal to the consultation exercise upon which it was based. Indeed, many of us in the development group are trainers. As MAP has gained from the experience of trainers, I hope it may contribute something to the improvement of vocational training. This may involve the clearer definition of what the requirements for trainers and their practices actually mean.

It is noteworthy how closely the two sets of criteria are aligned. There are only four JCPTGP criteria which MAP does not cover to some degree at least:

1   good-quality practice premises
2   an appropriate level of computerisation of records with systems that meet with NHS approval; computer use should be integrated into consultations
3   a practice library and other teaching aids, including a balance for the GP registrar between the gaining of clinical experience and other opportunities for learning
4   a sensitivity to the personal needs and feelings of colleagues.

Practice premises and computerisation are not assessed because MAP aims to include non-principals, who may well have no influence over buildings or computers. The education of registrars is not the responsibility of all MAP candidates. However, perhaps we should ask colleagues about the candidate's sensitivity towards others.

The MAP office opened to applications in April 1999, and the level of interest from all parts of the UK has been very encouraging. The first candidates are expected to complete the MAP requirements successfully during late 2000. I hope that the overlap between MAP standards and those for trainers and their practices will encourage doctors in training practices who are not yet College members to seriously consider whether they should offer themselves to peer assessment in this way. They could possibly even fulfil the requirements for revalidation at the same time.

References

1   Holden J and Wearne J (2000) Membership by assessment of performance: developing a method for assessing established general practitioners. *Br J Gen Pract.* **50**: 231–5.

2   Royal College of General Practitioners (2000) *Membership by Assessment of Performance. The MAP Handbook.* Royal College of General Practitioners, London.

3   Joint Committee on Postgraduate Training for General Practice (1998) *Recommendations to Deaneries on the Selection and Re-selection of General Practice Trainers.* Joint Committee on Postgraduate Training for General Practice, London.

Further details

Further information on MAP is available from:
   The MAP Administrator
   Royal College of General Practitioners
   14 Princes Gate
   Hyde Park
   London SW7 1PU.

Part 8

Supporting poorly performing doctors

The newspapers have been full of stories of poor clinical performance in both primary and secondary care. The notable cases of Mr Rodney Ledward and Harold Shipman have focused the public's attention on the medical profession as never before. The public no longer appears to have confidence in the medical profession's self-regulation in general and in the General Medical Council in particular. The recognition of poorly performing general practitioners is difficult because of their independent contractor status, but in recent years health authorities have begun to put in place procedures for identifying poorly performing general practitioners across the UK. These procedures are designed to identify the GP's poor performance at an early stage before a referral to the General Medical Council is required. It is important therefore that there are also mechanisms in place to support those doctors whose performance is not acceptable.

In this part of the book, Reed Bowden describes the need to support poorly performing doctors and introduces the concept of the local support group, but first John Skelton and his colleagues at the University of Birmingham describe in some detail mechanisms that they have developed to improve the communication skills of doctors both in training and in established practice.

35

Improving the communication skills of poorly performing doctors

John Skelton, Phil Croft, Connie Wiskin and Katharine Messenger

Introduction

Nowadays, communication skills are perceived as being 'core' parts of the undergraduate curriculum, and as 'core skills' for qualified doctors.[1,2] In the present climate, where vigilance about performance is seen to be central to the medical profession, it is clear that doctors are in principle as likely to be identified as having problems with communication as they are to be having problems with areas of clinical expertise. This in turn raises the question of what can be done to evaluate and support doctors who are so identified.

In the last two years it has become common in the West Midlands region for trainers (and, in general, more senior doctors) to be aware of the possibility that the problems which doctors appear to be experiencing may be due to poor communication. It is now becoming increasingly routine for such doctors to be referred to the Interactive Skills Unit (ISU) of the Department of Primary Care and General Practice at the University of Birmingham. The ISU specialises in the delivery of communication skills training and assessment for health professionals. It is a multidisciplinary team (team members have backgrounds in language, education and theatre as well as clinical medicine) which has acted as an educational resource, undertaking direct teaching, consultancy and teacher training both in the region and beyond.

This chapter will look at issues which arise from the referred doctors programme (so called to avoid the very negative connotations of the phrase 'poorly performing'), and at the issues that were raised during the workshop that we ran. Basic details of the referred doctors are described in Table 35.1. It will be seen from the table that the majority of our referrals come through

Table 35.1:   Details of referred doctors

General practitioners	9
Hospital doctors	17
Native speakers of English	5
Non-native speakers of English	21
UK qualified	8
Total (to October 2000)	26

Note: the total excludes two doctors who have been referred, but who have declined to attend.

Four of the 26 doctors have been UK citizens, UK qualified, Caucasian and native speakers of English.

the hospital system. However, unless the context makes the contrary clear, the points made below are equally applicable to hospital doctors and GPs.

For GPs there are two typical routes for referral. First, a GP may be identified as a result of failing the summative assessment examination at the end of the registrar year. In such cases the need for referral is clearly understood by the GP, and is well accepted. That is to say, the summative assessment examination seems to be accepted as a more or less fair test of the GP. This is the only group of doctors, either from general practice or from the hospital sector, that reaches us as a result of an external, researched assessment. Other doctors are referred either by the GMC on the basis of the (necessarily subjective) views of patients who are dissatisfied with their performance, or they come after having received one or more negative assessments by peers, superiors or patients in the hospital system. This means that these other doctors tend to come with a sense of grievance.

The referral process

When a doctor is referred to us, the typical procedure we undertake is as follows.

1   All appropriate and willing parties are contacted by telephone for discussion, and written documentation (where stakeholders are willing to release it) is gathered.
2   The doctor is interviewed by the Director of the ISU (JRS).
3   The interview with the doctor typically (but not always) concludes with an agreement for role-play training to be undertaken. This normally happens two or three weeks after the initial meeting. Role-plays are designed with the referred doctor him- or herself, often during the training and as part of it. We have learned that this gives us a great deal of understanding into how much insight and sophistication the doctor has when it comes

to communication in general and his or her own communication in particular. Role-plays are undertaken with two professional role-players and one academic present, and are followed by a detailed discussion. Training normally lasts two to three hours, and is exceptionally intensive.

4   One further possibility often arises during the training session, but is not really part of it. For reasons discussed below, many doctors are identified as having communication problems when the problem is in fact something else. It is sometimes necessary to address very directly with the doctor concerned other issues of his or her professional behaviour or attitude. The resultant discussion can be at best profound, and sometimes quite difficult for the doctor.

5   At the close of the training session, we have started to try to institute a formal OSCE-style evaluation of the doctor undertaking a role-play.

6   Finally, a written report is prepared for all interested parties.

From time to time there have been variations in this format. Sometimes we have not undertaken a role-play, and sometimes we have recommended, say, two afternoons of training. However, the above is the typical programme. One point which should be stressed is that we undertake to ensure that the whole process is entirely confidential (e.g. the training takes place on neutral territory away from the doctor's surgery and from the University Medical School) and we also undertake to share with the doctor concerned everything which we share with other stakeholders in the process. In particular, this means that we do not give one written report to the referred doctor and a somewhat different written report to those who may have the power to shape his or her career in the future.

It follows from the need for confidentiality that only a small number of academic and role-play staff can be involved in this work. Indeed, in addition to the routine training (which is in itself quite substantial) undertaken by members of the role-play team on making themselves available for ISU work, we offer additional training for work with the referred doctors. Role-players represent a range of professional backgrounds, tend to be degree educated, and are an integrated part of our curriculum teaching. To date, four of them have been trained for this work.

What are the key issues?

Is communication really the problem?

The problem is seldom quite as simple as this. That is to say, most referrals to us may have a communication problem as a common route (or perhaps more precisely a common label), but typically the problem is with communication and something else at the same time.

For example, a doctor who has switched from the hospital sector to the GP sector may not have fully professionalised him- or herself within a general practice context. He or she may therefore consult within a very medical model. This is a question of professional attitude rather than anything else and, as far as communication skills are concerned, what is at stake here may be little more than offering low-level routines (words, phrases, minor aspects of body language) which will facilitate a more holistic approach. However, the real issue often involves confirming to the doctor that this is indeed what is required.

Other doctors, particularly young doctors in the hospital sector, often give the impression that their problems stem from the fact that they are trying too hard to be (and present themselves as) efficient, on top of their work, precise and decisive. Such doctors often need merely to be offered the opportunity to talk about and construct an alternative professional persona. Indeed, with such doctors often the best advice one can offer is 'When you start your next rotation, try out a different professional self'.

For some doctors, particularly those who have qualified in the developing world, there may be issues of general education. Doctors may be accustomed to rote learning, and be poor at reflecting on their own performance as a consequence of this. They may not find it easy to organise and structure their consultations very effectively, and to the observer (and the patient) this creates a rather scatter-brained effect – and perhaps one reason for this is that they do not have a natural fluency of cognitive organisation. Other doctors may simply be generally very defensive when it comes to education, perhaps feeling that they might be somehow 'found out', and their lack of ability exposed to ridicule. In such cases doctors may react negatively to suggestions which are designed to be supportive.

Is race the issue?

A glance at Table 35.1 will reveal that the most striking feature of the doctors referred is the likelihood that they are not native-speaker Caucasians. There are a number of reasons why this might be so, ranging from the innocuous to the racist.

At the more innocuous end of the spectrum, one referral was of an African GP. We had observed him briefly on video (not a video submitted for summative assessment, to which non-clinical members of the team, rather exasperatingly, are denied access by the terms of the consent form which the patient signs). The doctor appeared to be very immobile and his consulting style was (apart from anything else) very dull. When we met him and worked with him face to face, it was clear that he had an unusually mobile and animated face, but this was entirely lost on video. Lighting black actors well is notoriously difficult, and it is quite possible that dark-skinned doctors are particularly vulnerable because the usually very imperfect circumstances under which their videos are made create additional problems for them which a light-skinned colleague would not experience. At the less innocuous end of the scale, it has to be said that a number of doctors come with a sense that their referral has a degree of racism attached to it. No GPs have yet claimed that this was a possibility.

Language has certainly been an issue with a number of referred doctors. This is because their command of English has not been particularly strong, or their accent has rendered them difficult to understand, or the cultural norms for speech in their own cultures are different to those which pertain in the UK. For example, we have had South-East Asian GPs referred to us who (perhaps principally because of the staccato delivery which is typical of their first languages) appear to be talking with a kind of machine-gun rapidity which is very likely to be misunderstood both by examiners looking at videos and by patients, and which therefore needs to be altered. The clearest example of this type of problem is perhaps the common perception in the UK that German speakers are somehow abrupt to the point of rudeness. This is simply a consequence of the natural phonological patterns of the German language, and the abruptness is entirely unintentional.

In the context of languages, it should be noticed that there is at present a serious anomaly. An Indian doctor who wishes to practise in this country may now expect to take a British Council English Language Test in India, and subsequently to take the Professional and Linguistic Assessment Board (PLAB) examination, which will include a communication skills element. There are no such expectations for a doctor who is a citizen of a European Union country. This is an important issue, particularly for general practice, which is a specialty in which good language and communication skills are at a premium. General practice is a very discursive area of medicine.

The stigma of poor performance

As we have already mentioned, GPs tend to find the verdict of the summative assessment examination fairly acceptable. It seems on the whole to be a less difficult label for them to bear than that of 'poor performance'. Doctors who are directly referred to us from one source or another as being 'poorly performing' tend to come with a much more defensive and resentful mind-set.

It is clear that if we are to support doctors who are having a problem then this ought, at least initially, to be in the context that we all have aspects of our professional performance which are not as good as we would wish them to be, and that it is the role of our trainers to draw attention to these areas and to help us to overcome the difficulties. As is always the case in teaching and train-ing, difficult truths should be rendered as palatable as possible by making them clear at an early stage. Bad news is made particularly unpleasant when it comes as a surprise.

What difference can you make in an afternoon?

As we go to press we have only evaluated the GP side of the referred doctors programme in detail. However, GP participants and their trainers do indicate that training appears to make a difference, although this is heavily qualified by the recognition that a great many people do a great many things to sup-port those who fail summative assessment.

It is important to bear in mind here that often an improvement in com-munication skills is not entirely the point. A normally intelligent and insight-ful doctor who has a blind spot (e.g. about how he or she is perceived by colleagues) can have this difficulty removed in an afternoon. A doctor who is generally good at communication and has been unlucky enough to be referred is likely to improve radically simply by having his or her good qualities con-firmed. A doctor who has been quietly aware for some time of problems will respond massively when these problems are taken seriously and addressed seriously, and so on. However, we certainly would not claim that we can make a radical improvement in every case. Again, precisely because communication on its own is not really what is at stake, we are faced with the difficult truth in one or two cases that people who are not well suited to medicine generally may end up with us because there is nowhere else to send them.

Can you assess them in a single afternoon?

We assess doctors partly on the basis of an afternoon's training, partly on the preliminary interview conducted with the Director, and partly on any shared documentation and other views that we receive. It is, of course, true that doctors are on their best behaviour when they meet us – they would be extremely foolish if they were not. And it is notoriously difficult to assess attitudes by observing performance. The other events which occur around the training, and particularly the way in which doctors discuss and build up with us role-play scenarios which they then undertake, give us some insight into some aspects of their attitude. However, it would not always be easy for us to identify, for example, a habit of arrogance which the doctor was capable of suppressing on particular occasions (although an accusation of arrogance by a stakeholder – which we have had – is taken very seriously, and role-plays are identified to deal with it). We are only now beginning to explore the possibility of some type of formal assessment towards the end of the training session. At present it is not clear to us how much this would add to the very detailed report which gets written, but we are conscious of the sometimes very high stakes that are involved, and we wish to do our best by the public in the first instance and the doctor in the second.

Conclusion

This kind of work is probably here to stay. The little evidence that we have to date suggests that direct, intensive training of this type performs a useful function, with a number of stakeholders voicing the view that it should be made available to everyone, perhaps as part of the re-accreditation process.

However, one main advantage that it has – and this is an advantage about which it is possible to be equivocal – is that we offer a locus of teaching for doctors with a wide range of troubling non-clinical problems. This is obviously a good thing in the sense that some training is better than none, but it does mean that a wide range of concerns and difficulties are repackaged as 'communication problems'.

References

1   General Medical Council (1993) *Tomorrow's Doctors*. General Medical Council, London.

2   British Medical Association (1998) *Communication Skills and Continuing Professional Development*. British Medical Association, London.

36

First aid for the poorly performing doctor

Reed Bowden

The General Medical Council (GMC), which has always had mechanisms for dealing with appalling performance and for doctors whose work was affected by illness, introduced performance procedures for persistently poor work in July 1997. These procedures are based in law.

Parallel local procedures via health authorities were brought in at the same time. They are based in regulation, and mediated through the health authorities' Quality in Practice initiatives. They are intended for underperformance of a lesser degree, and are also used for the remediation of doctors who have already been seen by the GMC and suspended, or whose registration has been made conditional.

The local support group

Many health authorities now have local support groups (their names vary), and the details both of the factors that trigger their activities, and of their procedures, may differ. All of them are based on the ScHARR report (School of Health and Related Research, Sheffield University, September 1997).

The health authority triggers the process, but in a few cases it is delegated to the primary care groups (PCGs). Triggering factors might be repeated complaints from patients, whistleblowing by other doctors or by employed or attached staff, or complaints from hospital departments. Poor performance indicators such as PGEA non-attendance, or failure to achieve targets such as cervical smear levels, provide another clue. There is also a subgroup where the GMC have considered official complaints and believe that local procedures will suffice. The triggering factors must be multiple, well-founded and attested.

Typically, the local support group has five members – two health authority representatives, two from the local medical committee (LMC) and a deanery educationalist. In any particular case, a working subgroup of one/one/one is formed. Often the LMC representative will attend just the early meetings, and then the others will carry them forward. The membership of the committees and working subgroups is still evolving and may vary in the future.

The typical clients are often single-handed practitioners. If they are in partnership, the whole practice may be struggling, or just one partner. Most are men. They tend to be aged 55 years or older, and have qualified abroad. They often work in tough deprived areas, and their communication skills are usually poor.

The visiting process

The first step is to arrange a visit. A letter and telephone call from the local support group to the client inform them that concerns have arisen, but the sources are not identified. The letter emphasises the wish to help, not condemn, and the intention to make more formal procedures unnecessary. At the first visit, the visitors stress two points, namely that patient care and safety are paramount, and that we must all try to meet the requirements of the GMC's booklets *Good Medical Practice* and *Maintaining Good Medical Practice*. The doctor(s) and key staff are interviewed and the premises are toured. The visitors try to be alert to structural and other problems with the premises, and to possible health issues. Subsequent visits are made in order to learn more and develop relationships until a structured report can be negotiated. Eventually the report is rewritten as a plan for improvement, with a timescale attached to each subsection. Education is always part of this plan.

Drawbacks to the system

The investigative methods are strong on face validity but weak on objectivity and reliability. The visitors are viewed as policemen, not helpers, so visits may be tolerated because the only further step is formal referral to the GMC. Another drawback is that the GMC can be unrealistic in their judgement of what local procedures can achieve.

Client factors against success

These include denial of problems, or of continuing problems, and denial of the facts. They may believe that it is all someone else's fault. Typically there is ignorance (often profound) of educational methods or importance. The clients may show unreliability with regard to attending meetings and meeting dead-lines. They do not always see the possible pathway towards formal procedures and loss of registration.

The future

Some PCG/PCTs are already bringing special concern groups into being, via their clinical governance subcommittees. These include lay representation. Some of us working in this field see the PCG as the natural setting for remediation. The details of revalidation are not yet definite, but we know that it will involve local profiling, to include educational personal development plans and practice personal development plans as well as target-reaching and other matters. This should identify poor performers and raise the possibility of helping them via the clinical governance mechanism of their PCG, possibly by using protocols, mentors and inter-practice co-operation. There is also a general perception that the GMC is getting tougher in response to public, governmental and professional pressure, and in the light of a number of high-profile cases of under-performance in the recent past. This could reduce the number of doctors who are referred back by the GMC for local help, many of whom seem to be beyond local (or perhaps any) remediation.

Postscript: the UKCRA workshop

The workshop produced the following suggestions (in no particular order of importance).

The performance indicators method of assessing performance, previously thought to correlate poorly with actual performance, now seems to be giving a truer picture. One system is that pioneered in Rotherham. The data that make up a Rotherham profile are for the most part publicly available, and all heath authorities could easily collect them if they are not doing so already.

There was some support for trying to separate the organisational elements of poor performance from personal factors. The PCGs/PCTs were seen as the proper bodies to assess systems, and local performance committees for the personal factors, but in practice it might be impossible to separate them in this way. PCG personnel might be prejudiced if they were asked to investigate a doctor from their own group.

Some workshop members saw benefits in separating assessment from support. This is the subject of widespread debate at the moment. It may be possible to use the expertise of the lay members of the present Independent Review Tribunals, which will soon be phased out. They could (perhaps with some extra training) be asked to join the local support groups' assessment visits.

There was regret that Professor Lesley Southgate's formal GMC assessment procedures could not be made available to local groups, although the reasons (chiefly degradation of the tool by widespread dissemination of its contents, and also copyright issues) were understood. We thought that other simulation groups might be used, namely the Leicester or Leeds groups, or Peter Burrows' MRCGP group. Another possibility was the use (with prior consent) of 'masked patients'.

Some advocated wider membership of support groups, perhaps to be renamed quality groups, with increased lay representation (*see* above), and also members from the Overseas Doctors Association in areas where many clients were from overseas.

We felt that the educational prescription, which would always form part of the overall help offered, should be built round PDPs, PPDPs and auditing.

There was also the hope that the annual appraisals that will form part of revalidation will also provide an early warning sign of doctors who are beginning to struggle in their work, so that remedies can be offered in good time.

Part 9

Clinical governance

Clinical governance was defined in the Department of Health (1998) publication, *A First-Class Service: Quality in the New NHS*, as 'offering work through which NHS organisations are accountable for continuously improving the quality of their services and safeguarding the high standards of care ... creating an environment in which excellence in clinical care will flourish'. It is therefore essentially a concept which involves organisations. It is a concept for the whole of the NHS, which involves learning from mistakes and failures and spreading good practice, and it is a powerful mechanism for improving the quality of care provided to our patients.

In this part of the general practice jigsaw, Guy Houghton, Clinical Director of the renowned Birmingham Health Authority Clinical Governance Support Unit, introduces the concepts of clinical governance in primary care, and presents the findings of a research project which focused on the new clinical governance leads of the 61 primary care groups in the West Midlands. The prolific authors and educationalists Ruth Chambers and Jill Wakley then describe the process and outcomes of workshops that they have organised in Staffordshire which have helped to produce the culture of clinical governance in primary care groups.

37

The introduction of clinical governance in primary care: teaching and learning needs

Guy Houghton

The concept of clinical governance was first introduced in *The New NHS: Modern, Dependable*.[1] It was intended as a part of the latest NHS reforms to emphasise the need for individual and organisational accountability for quality in the service. Along with professional self-regulation and lifelong learning, it was designed to form the basis of the personal and professional development of all staff working in the NHS. Initially the White Paper defined clinical governance in terms of ten elements or attributes of a quality organisation. These ten elements are listed in Table 37.1.

Table 37.1: The elements of clinical governance

- Quality improvement (including clinical audit)
- Leadership
- Evidence-based practice
- Dissemination of good practice, ideas and innovation
- Clinical risk reduction
- Detection of adverse events
- Learning lessons from complaints
- Addressing poor clinical performance
- Professional development programmes
- High-quality data

Although the White Paper provided a conceptual framework, the actual practical implications and expectations were not spelled out until the publication in March 1999 of the Health Service Circular *Clinical Governance: Quality in the New NHS*, less than a month before the new primary care groups (PCGs) took up their responsibilities.[2] As well as preparing themselves for their new central role in the NHS reorganisation with all of the other tasks devolved to them, the PCG boards had to identify a clinical governance lead to take responsibility for improving the standards of practice and quality of care of all practitioners in the locality with little appreciation of what would be required of them. It was anticipated that each practice would then nominate a clinical governance lead who would reflect at practice level the quality agenda set by the PCG.

This meant that these clinical governance leads – local practitioners initially elected to the PCG board by their peers and then selected by the board – would have the responsibility for all quality initiatives throughout the PCG, at the same time as ensuring that practices understood the whole concept of clinical governance and its practical implications. With the guidance only available three weeks before the start of the entire PCG reorganisation, there was understandable concern that the clinical governance leads might lack the knowledge, skills and understanding necessary for the task.

Clinical governance leads in the West Midlands

As a start, in the West Midlands it was decided to survey the experience and expertise of the leads and their perceived educational needs. The results of this survey have been published in detail in the *Journal of Clinical Governance*.[3]

A questionnaire was sent to all of the identified clinical governance leads in the 61 primary care groups in the West Midlands. The questions asked about higher qualifications, educational appointments and training, experience in representing peers at local medical committee and health authority level, involvement with clinical audit, and the strengths that each individual felt he or she brought to the role.

The educational needs assessment involved each individual ranking the ten elements of clinical governance (as shown in Table 37.1) on a numerical scale according to their perceived training need. Each individual was asked to state their personal preferences with regard to the style, provision, timing and venue of possible educational events.

In total, 57 out of a possible 63 questionnaires were returned. At this time four PCGs had not yet appointed a clinical governance lead and several had joint appointments. A total of 51 general practitioners and 6 nurses replied.

It was found that 48% of GPs held the MRCGP, proportionally equivalent to the work-force. Only two FRCGPs were involved as clinical governance leads. Ten individuals had been GP tutors and six had been VTS course organisers (altogether less than one-third of the leads). The only teaching in educational method had been attendance at a GP trainers' course (22 out of 51), again representing less than half of the leads. One-third had been on their local medical audit advisory group and one-third had LMC experience.

There were 44 male and 7 female responders. All of them had been qualified for at least ten years. There was a diverse range of backgrounds, with 17 responders qualifying from Birmingham (the local medical school), seven from Oxford or Cambridge, six from India, six from London, ten from other English universities, two from Ireland and one from Africa.

In terms of educational provision, a range of teaching styles and learning experiences and opportunities were desired, with a particular need for training in change management techniques. The training requirements relating to the ten specific elements of clinical governance were ranked in the following order (*see* Table 37.2).

Table 37.2: Ten+ elements of clinical governance (in descending order of educational need according to Likert scale mean score)

Element of clinical governance	Number giving score					Mean score
	1	*2*	*3*	*4*	*5*	
Tackling poor performance	2	1	7	20	20	4.1
Leadership skills	1	1	11	19	18	4.0
Building on good practice	0	2	14	17	17	4.0
High-quality data	1	3	13	14	19	3.9
Clinical risk reduction	1	3	11	20	15	3.9
Professional development programmes	2	2	12	20	13	3.8
Significant event analysis	0	6	12	18	14	3.8
Evidence-based practice	1	4	13	19	13	3.8
Quality assurance	2	2	14	19	13	3.8
Clinical audit	2	6	11	16	14	3.7
Learning from complaints	0	8	17	17	7	3.5

The number of non-responses ranged between 7 and 8.

The survey led to the following rather unsatisfactory conclusions. No attributes were consistently demonstrated as underpinning the selection of clinical governance leads. Free-text analysis suggested personal enthusiasm ranging from evangelical zeal to improve quality to pressganged 'volunteers'. The lack of an explicit explanation of what would be expected of the clinical governance leads at the time of their appointment, in conjunction with a lack of prior training for PCGs, had not helped the selection process. Training would have to be undertaken at the same time as learning through experience in a new role without compromising practice commitments and patient care.

Facilitating clinical governance: using a clinical governance support unit

In Birmingham we adopted the model of a clinical governance support unit to assist PCGs, which in its remit included a monthly meeting for all PCG clinical governance leads in the city to provide training in the different aspects of clinical governance.[4] The original Birmingham medical audit advisory group (MAAG) had evolved over the years from the initial facilitation of medical (and later clinical) audit activities to offering clinical effectiveness training.[5] The introduction of clinical governance expanded the triad of clinical audit, clinical guidelines and evidence-based practice by incorporating these into a wider process based on the themes of:

- responsibility and accountability
- comprehensive quality improvement
- risk management
- identification of poor performance.[6]

Birmingham Health Authority appreciated that PCGs and their clinical governance leads needed some central direction and co-ordination, and allowed the MAAG to develop into a clinical governance support unit.[7]

In the first year, the clinical governance leads have had presentations and training to include sessions on the following:

- poorly performing practitioners – from Dr Alistair Short, based on his experience with the pilot scheme in Glasgow
- clinical risk reduction – from the Medical Defence Union
- an introduction to personal learning plans – from Dr Steve Field, the West Midlands Regional Director of Postgraduate General Practice Education
- the requirements of the Caldicott Report on issues of confidentiality in the use of data.

These presentations cover four of the top six topics identified as learning needs by the clinical governance leads region-wide. Leadership as such scarcely lends itself to the subject of a tutorial, although the skills required to effect change management may well need to be explored and rehearsed. The monthly meeting in itself provides a forum for the exchange of views and experiences, so that all of the PCGs in the city can be encouraged to learn from their neighbours – from both successful and less fortunate initiatives.

References

1   Department of Health (1997) *The New NHS: Modern, Dependable*. Department of Health, London.

2   NHS Executive (1999) *Health Service Circular 1999/065. Clinical Governance in the New NHS*. NHS Executive, London.

3   Houghton G, Wall D and Field S (1999) Primary care group clinical governance leads: their educational needs and experiences. *J Clin Govern*. **7**: 190–4.

4   Houghton G, Taylor S and Fraser J (2000) Role of a clinical governance unit in primary care (abstract). *J Integ Care*. **4**: 56–7.

5   Houghton G and Sproston B (1998) Clinical effectiveness: the new challenge for MAAGs. *Audit Trends*. **6**: 50–3.

6   Houghton G and Wall D (2000) Twelve tips on teaching about clinical governance. *Med Teacher*. **22**: 145–53.

7   Sproston B and Houghton G (1998) Clinical governance: the future for MAAGs. *Audit Trends*. **6**: 86–9.

38

How can you teach GPs and primary care professionals to adopt the culture of clinical governance? Try the Staffordshire University way!

Ruth Chambers and Gill Wakley

You have to engage and involve GPs and primary care professionals, to help them to decide that they must embrace a change of culture in their workplace, before you can show them how to apply clinical governance in practice.

Running more than 20 workshops to teach GPs, nurses, therapists and non-clinical staff working in primary and community care about clinical governance has convinced us that participants need time to reflect on the new information they have experienced in the workshop or other learning event – both during that educational session and afterwards while they are planning what to do.

At Staffordshire University we provide workshops for a mix of 12 to 20 professionals, who may be individuals attending on their own, or several people who work together in a general practice or a department within the directorate of a community trust. The facilitators are multidisciplinary, too.

The aims of the workshops are as follows:

1   to increase the participants' understanding of the meaning and application of clinical governance
2   to increase the participants' understanding of how clinical governance may be meaningfully developed in various workplace settings
3   to agree a priority area and develop a timetabled action plan with other colleagues in the workplace that incorporates the principles of best practice in clinical governance.

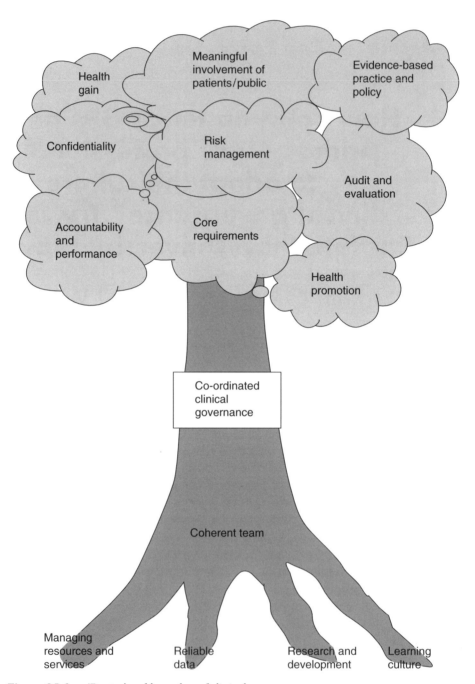

Figure 38.1: 'Routes' and branches of clinical governance.

The intended outcomes of the workshop are as follows:

1 that participants should understand the meaning, principles of best practice, and application of clinical governance
2 that participants should have constructed a framework for a timetabled action plan to apply clinical governance in their workplace.

The definition of clinical governance that we use is about 'implementing care that works in an environment in which clinical effectiveness can flourish within a facilitatory culture'.[1] We elicit the components of clinical governance from the audience, using our home-made diagram of the clinical governance 'tree' (*see* Figure 38.1) to point out any missing components. The audience usually omits such aspects of clinical governance as 'confidentiality', 'health gains' and 'meaningful involvement of patients and the public in planning and delivering healthcare', and focuses on components such as 'evidence-based care', 'audit and evaluation' and 'accountability'. The ensuing discussion about the importance of all of these components increases awareness of the interrelationship of organisational and clinical aspects of clinical governance, and helps the non-clinical attendees to recognise the part they have to play in applying clinical governance in practice.

Short presentations by well-informed GP and practice nurse speakers to the workshop delegates describe practical examples of how to apply clinical governance in practice around clinically important topics such as asthma and diabetes, and organisational topics such as risk management or reliable and accurate data.

Much of the workshop time is given over to small group work whereby participants work together to draft protocols for clinical governance programmes to take back to their workplaces. The final plenary discussion of draft clinical governance plans allows participants to refine their draft protocols in the light of others' constructive comments. The delegates are encouraged to agree those draft protocols with their managers and work colleagues, drawing in as many colleagues as possible to the programme and seeking managers' support and comments as appropriate. The finalised protocols are posted back to the workshop facilitators, who provide personal written feedback within a week.

Box 38.1:   Clinical governance protocol used in the workshop

1   Select a priority topic. Please write out the title.
   • Why did you choose this topic?
   • Is it a priority area? (Yes/No)
   If yes, whose priority is it? Please circle all that apply. Practice/district health improvement programme/government/district health issue/the PCG/PCT/the trust/the health authority/patients/community/workplace colleagues/self/professional/subject of national service framework/subject of

continued overleaf

National Institute for Clinical Excellence/previous or recent significant event (organisational, clinical or performance)/other (please specify).

- What problem are you addressing?
- What changes do you hope to make?
- How did you choose the topic? Please circle all that apply.

By consensus in discussion with others/I decided on behalf of my work colleagues/my practice, PCG/PCT or trust requested the topic/looked at others' strategic plan/manager's recommendation/patient or carer's request/ other (please specify).

2   What will you do? Please tick the relevant items in the list below. Try to en-sure that you include as many of the principles of good practice in clinical governance as possible, which are to:

- include multidisciplinary input
- address national, local, organisational or professional priorities
- involve partnership working (e.g. between agencies, or between man-agement and clinicians)
- incorporate input from patients (e.g. user, carer, the public; at training, planning, monitoring or delivery stages)
- be capable of achieving health gains
- be based on evidence-based practice, policy or management
- incorporate input and commitment from managers to enable action to take place (e.g. protected time for staff involved)
- demonstrate standards and achievements.

2.1 Who will lead the clinical governance programme? Please circle.
Doctor/nurse/manager/other (please specify)

- Who else will be involved?

2.2 Who will do what?

2.3 What data or information will you gather?

- At baseline
- After intervention or change in services or practice.

2.4 How will you involve patients or the general public, when, and at what stage?

2.5 When will you start? What is the timetable?

2.6 What do you expect to achieve?

- What specific outcomes do you expect?
- How will you measure them?
- How can you demonstrate any improvements or changes from the baseline where you are now to anyone, or to us as facilitators?

2.7 What help will you want from the following?

- The management
- The library
- Us as facilitators?

This initiative is still relatively new, but so far about 25% of those attending have reported significant changes in practice to the facilitators six months or so after the workshops were held. These changes range from improving clinical practice by identifying and rectifying shortfalls in best practice (as an extension of clinical audit by involving patients and the public, and other partners or disciplines in providing care) to arranging for the school nurse to have a drawer and a share of a desk in a general practice as a result of close teamworking to bring the enuresis service for children into the surgery (resulting in all sorts of other spin-offs in multidisciplinary, cross-sector working in other areas of children's healthcare).

We have written a clinical governance workbook entitled *How to Do It* for any staff working at the community trust. The first 500 copies have been snapped up, and the workbook is currently being reprinted for other staff working there. Some of the members of the executive of the trust contributed short paragraphs which helped to individualise the workbook. The management have welcomed and endorsed the workbook as a sensible way to approach the application of clinical governance across the trust. The staff like having a tangible workbook that has helped to organise clinical governance into manageable components, made it relevant to everyday work, and allowed those using the programme to acknowledge what they are already doing well, and build upon their success.

The funding for the venture and the workbooks for the community trusts came from Staffordshire and Shropshire Non-Medical Educational Consortium. The workshops and subsequent work with primary care groups were commissioned by the health authority on behalf of the five PCGs in their district.

The workshop at the UKCRA conference centred on a game to involve the participants in learning about planning for clinical governance in an interactive way (*see* Box 38.1). The lessons that emerged from the UKCRA workshop in learning about clinical governance as GPs, other health professionals or non-clinical support staff are that you need the following:

- very focused, timetabled planning if you are to involve all of the team in a clinical governance programme
- a multidisciplinary approach (GPs, practice-employed and attached staff), with everyone's roles and responsibilities made clear
- participants to accept that quality is everyone's business
- to involve others from outside your workplace (e.g. leisure, sports, education, local government, etc.)
- to try to adopt a priority for your team which overlaps with the priorities between government, district, primary care organisation (PCO), practice and practitioner

- to find out about patients' views and act on them (e.g. involve patients in training, if feedback from patients in general has indicated that the staff have specific learning needs)
- to overcome barriers to multidisciplinary working
- to know where to seek information about priority areas (population statistics, etc.)
- good communication and good information-gathering/exchange for coherent planning
- a learning culture in your workplace.

You can read more about this topic and approach on www.primarycare online.co.uk.

Reference

1   Chambers R and Wakley G (2000) *Making Clinical Governance Work for You.* Radcliffe Medical Press, Oxford.

Part 10

Revalidation

Patients must be able to trust doctors with their lives and well-being. To justify that trust, we as a profession have a duty to maintain a good standard of practice and care and to show respect for human life.

The General Medical Council used these words in the introduction to its excellent booklet, *Good Medical Practice*.[1] This booklet has become the bedrock of both clinical governance and the future system of revalidation. While clinical governance will ensure consistency of healthcare across the UK, revalidation will involve a periodic assessment of individual doctors, to ensure that doctors who are not fit to practise will be discovered, made subject to conditions, suspended or removed from the register. It will be a transparent system that will ensure patients are not at risk from poorly performing doctors.

The General Medical Council is consulting widely, and the Royal Colleges and other professional groups are involved in discussions which will lead to a process that should in turn lead to the introduction of the system in 2002.

This part of the book has been written by general practitioners who are actively engaged in the development of revalidation processes, to cast light on the consultation process and also raise a number of important questions. They give us valuable insights into what is going to affect us all in the very near future.

References

1   General Medical Council (1998) *Good Medical Practice*. General Medical Council, London.

39

Revalidation for general practice

Mike Pringle and Terry Bradley

Introduction

In the words of the General Medical Council,[1] 'patients trust doctors with their lives and well-being. They need to have confidence that their doctor is competent and abides by high ethical standards.' Although the vast majority of doctors meet this expectation, recent cases of serious clinical failure confirm the need for reform.

The concept of some form of reassessment of doctors is not new, and there have been a number of attempts in recent years by the professional bodies within general practice to describe a model for the previous attempts. However, they have failed to deliver it. The difference now is that all of the major professional bodies are committed to delivering revalidation and the government appears to be willing to resource the infrastructure necessary for some important aspects of the process.

All of the Colleges have been asked to describe a mechanism for revalidation. The Royal College of General Practitioners (RCGP) working party has been resourced by the college but has representation from the General Practitioners Committee, the Overseas Doctors Association, the National Association of Non-Principals, the Committee of General Practice Education Directors (COGPED), the National Association of General Practice Tutors (NAGPT), the Small Practice Association, the General Medical Council (GMC) and patient representatives.

Revalidation: a continuous process, not an event

Although the cycle of revalidation will be five years, it must be understood that this interval is too long for two reasons. First, it would obviously be totally unacceptable to patients and the public to permit unsafe practice to go unchecked for this length of time. Secondly, it would be undesirable for a GP to suddenly find him- or herself unable to practise when it may well be that remedial action taken sufficiently early could correct shortfalls satisfactorily.

The revalidation system

Appraisal

All general practitioners will be required to collect a portfolio of evidence throughout the five-year cycle. They will be visited annually by a trained general practitioner who will assess and appraise them in their progress towards lifelong learning, and check that they are on track for revalidation.

A folder of material (as described below) is then submitted to a local revalidation committee. At present it would appear that there would be one committee each for Scotland and Wales. The number in England is as yet undetermined, but it could be one per region.

Three people will assess each application:

• a general practitioner who knows the general practitioner being assessed and his or her practice area
• a 'distant' general practitioner
• a lay person.

It is likely that for 90–95% of applications the submission will be approved and a letter written to the GMC recommending the doctor for revalidation. For those who fail the process or come to the light of the committee via another route, or for those who do not fully understand the material, a practice visit will be offered. However, in the event of a query about a doctor's health it may be more appropriate to offer an occupational health consultation.

General practitioners who default from the process will be offered support to help them to achieve the standards required for revalidation. This could take the form of specific educational interventions arranged by postgraduate deaneries or occupational health supports. If a doctor fails to respond to supports offered or declines offers of support, he or she will in the last analysis be referred to the GMC, but it must be emphasised that this process is about revalidation, not devalidation.

Resources

With approximately 32 000 general practitioners needing to be appraised every year, it is clear that substantial resources will have to be devoted to this process. The Secretary of Health has stated that annual appraisals will take place.[2] However, if the Government does not fund annual appraisals then they simply will not happen. Assuming that annual appraisal is funded and does take place, it is estimated that it will be necessary, in the view of the RCGP, to employ one full-time equivalent (fte) assessor for every 50 general practitioners. For example, a practice with four doctors would have an annual visit, the assessor spending approximately half a day examining the general practitioners' professional development plans, audits and the complaints procedure. Time would be spent on discussions of plans for personal and practice development. It seems likely that this process will be run by the postgraduate deaneries.

The gold standard

The process described above begs the question of what it is that general practitioner will be judged against. *Good Medical Practice for General Practitioners*[3] was adapted from *Good Medical Practice*[4] by a working party led by Professor Martin Roland. Criteria were described for an 'excellent' general practitioner as well as for an unacceptable general practitioner. In total, 40 000 copies of the document were circulated to the profession in December 1999, and the document was supported by 15 to 1. In the light of helpful comments, a further version is being drafted. As a follow-up to *Good Medical Practice for General Practitioners*, a practical guide to the process has been developed. This is called *Criteria, Standards and Evidence*, and it will set out in detail what is expected of every general practitioner in the UK.

The first question to be answered by the doctor is 'Are you in clinical general practice?' If the answer to this question is yes, then all of the criteria for clinical general practice must be met. If the doctor also has other commitments (e.g. teaching, research or medical management) then there will be three key questions.

- How do you know you are competent to do the job described?
- What are you doing to update your skills?
- Who is your appraiser and where is the evidence that you have been appraised?

For example, a general practitioner trainer will need to say how they acquired their teaching skills, how they are keeping their training skills up to date, and whether they have been appraised. A university lecturer who currently undergoes an appraisal every two years will need to have this annually and produce evidence of it. Similar regulations will apply to clinical procedures which are not usually core to general practitioners' work (e.g. colposcopy).

It is clear that because this is a new system, some problems may become apparent during its introduction. Steps will be taken to ensure that there is no systematic discrimination against any one group of doctors because of their location, patient mix, practice size, etc.

What evidence must clinical GPs submit?

The results of appraisal must be submitted with a statement by the appraiser that in each year the applicant was on track for revalidation. In addition, general practitioners will be required to submit markers of performance on a number of dimensions of professional practice. These will include the following.

1 A requirement to read *Good Medical Practice for General Practitioners* and to sign a global declaration that they do not match the description of an unacceptable general practitioner as defined in any of the criteria listed in the document.

2 *Communication skills.* The proposed inclusion of this criterion generated many debates in the working group. It was finally agreed to include it because over half of all complaints against GPs are about communication.[5] This is the only area where general practitioners will be asked to collect evidence that they will not be gathering for another purpose (e.g. clinical governance or a personal development plan). The minimum action needed to fulfil this requirement will be a patient satisfaction questionnaire completed by at least 50 patients (e.g. John Howie's empowerment questionnaire).[6] Other options include videotapes of consultations or simulated surgeries, but with 32 000 GPs involved, the chosen method must be practicable. It will ultimately be possible to develop norms and acceptable levels for whatever method is chosen. The rigour and independence of the procedure must be demonstrable.

3 *Complaints procedure and critical incidents.* General practitioners must demonstrate that they have a complaints procedure in place, and show the actual complaints made annually and how they have responded to these. The nature of the complaints forms part of the process of triangulation. For example, if a general practitioner has had five complaints about rudeness or their communication skills, this would help to build up a picture of the practitioner. It appears from early experiences that underperforming GPs show deficiencies across a whole range of different dimensions of practice.

4 *Continuing professional development.* General practitioners will be required to submit a portfolio of evidence of reflective practice, responding to educational needs, evidence of improvement and participation in appropriate local combined audit.

5 *Access.* General practitioners will be required to outline their hours of availability such as are already described in practice leaflets, on websites, etc.

6   *Medical records.* The standard required is that another doctor taking over the care of that patient should be able to understand the patient's history and be able to take over their care on the basis of the notes. It has been suggested that 50 records should be sampled, but the practicalities of this are recognised, and work is ongoing to determine the optimum number required for this process.

7   *Annual appraisal.* This has been described above.

8   *Utilisation of resources.* Data on prescribing and referral will be collected by the general practitioner's primary care group or trust. While there is debate about what constitutes good referral practice,[7] doctors will be given the opportunity to explain highly unusual patterns, given their practice and patient profile.

Some common questions

1   *Will general practitioners be given protected time to prepare material for revalidation?* It seems likely that considerable resources will be required for the infrastructure for the process. There is concern that there is time built into the consultant contract for quality processes, but that this does not apply to the general practitioner's contract. It seems likely that the profession will need to continue to apply for protected time for quality initiatives such as this.

2   *Will the revalidation panel collect information locally about the practice?* This would not usually be necessary, but where questions have been raised about the practice, the local revalidation panel may choose to send out, say, 15 questionnaires to individuals such as the pharmacist, the district nurse, the local medical committee (LMC) secretary and the PCG/PCT lead. What will be sought is a professional view of the doctor's performance. This information will supplement the information gathered from the other sources alluded to above. It should be made clear that lying about the declaration of compliance with good medical practice is a GMC offence.

3   *What is the relationship between revalidation and clinical governance structures?* The NHS has the right to ensure the quality of the systems of care, which is distinct from the way in which patients experience that care. Revalidation deals with the professional aspects of care as opposed to the systems of care. Clearly, however, it is essential that these processes work in a complementary manner.

4   *If a general practitioner fails to meet the minimum standards of revalidation, is it more desirable to have an 'empty seat' or to tolerate a poor standard of care?* Until recently it appeared to be better to have poor doctoring services than none at all. However, opinion seems to have changed recently, and it is now accepted that it is better to act promptly to upgrade skills or refer

appropriately than to have unacceptable practice. One offshoot of this process could well be to provide objective evidence of the need for more resources in particular areas in order to sustain good medical practice. Indeed a case can be made for special financial and educational incentives to attract new general practitioners to such areas.

5   *Will revalidation have special effects in deprived areas?* There is a real risk that some older doctors working in deprived areas may choose to retire rather than change to meet new standards. However, the standards are being written in such a way that all general practitioners should be able to meet them, regardless of the context in which they work. If the initial evidence that is submitted is inconclusive, a practice visit will look at performance in the context of the practice.

6   *Will the communication skills assessment be conducted in English only?* Communication skills assessments may need to be conducted in languages other than English.

7   *How will the local revalidation panels be constituted and trained?* The boards will consist of representatives of the lay population, the LMC, overseas doctors and non-principals. The GMC will fund the local revalidation committees. Their structure and functions will be described in detail in a forthcoming document on the subject. Some of these functions overlap with the 'quality and performance in the NHS clinical indicators'.[8]

8   *Will the assessors be GP tutors?* This is possible, but their role would be much wider than that which is currently undertaken by GP tutors. They will be involved in appraisal, professional development, career counselling and measuring quality assurance. It is possible that people who are not general practitioners could be appointed to these posts, but whatever their background they must have the support and confidence of the profession.

Conclusion

The introduction of change on such a massive scale will undoubtedly be perceived as threatening by some professionals. However, there will be a range of benefits to patients, doctors and employers.

The GMC have described these as follows.

Benefits for the patient

These include:

*   protecting them from poorly performing doctors
*   promoting good medical practice

- making the register a valid indicator of current fitness to practise
- increasing their confidence in doctors.

Benefits for the doctors

These include:

- helping conscientious doctors to show that they are giving good medical care
- enabling doctors to correct weaknesses in their practice
- protecting doctors from unfounded criticisms of their fitness to practise.

Benefits for the employers

These include:

- providing the assurance and protection that will flow from knowing that the doctors whom they employ are fit to practise
- providing an additional mechanism to identify poor performance.

References

1   General Medical Council (2000) *Revalidating Doctors – Ensuring Standards, Securing the Future*. General Medical Council, London.

2   Department of Health (1999) *Supporting Doctors, Protecting Patients – a Consultation Paper on Preventing, Recognising and Dealing with Poor Clinical Performance of Doctors in the NHS in England*. Department of Health, London.

3   Royal College of General Practitioners (1999) *Good Medical Practice for General Practitioners – Draft for Consultation*. Royal College of General Practitioners, London.

4   General Medical Council (1998) *Good Medical Practice*. General Medical Council, London.

5   Meryn S (1998) Improving doctor–patient communication. *BMJ*. **316**: 1922–30.

6   Howie J, Heaney DJ, Maxwell M *et al.* (1999) Quality of general practice consultations: cross-sectional survey. *BMJ*. **319**: 738–43.

7   Wilkin D (1992) Patterns of referral: explaining variation. In: M Roland and A Coulter (eds) *Hospital Referrals*. Oxford University Press, Oxford.

8   Department of Health (1992) *NHS – Quality and Performance in the NHS: Clinical Indicators*. Department of Health, London.

40

Visions and problems

David Snadden

Revalidation is going to exercise us, both now, in terms of what it is going to be and how we will deliver it, and in the future, in terms of how it will affect us as a profession and personally. This brief report was written just as the General Medical Council (GMC) published their consultation document[1] on their revalidation proposals. Whatever the outcome of the GMC's consultation process, revalidation in one form or another will happen, and it will happen by 2002. The vision for revalidation seems on the surface straightforward enough. The proposed model consists of a five-year cycle, at the end of which every doctor will have to supply evidence that they remain fit to practise. This evidence will be collected under the headings set out by the GMC in their publication *Good Medical Practice*,[2] and will be reviewed annually at an appraisal. The evidence will be contained within a folder which will be submitted locally to a revalidation group that will decide whether the doctor should be revalidated or referred to the GMC fitness-to-practise procedures. The process will be externally reviewed to ensure that the decisions of the group meet national standards.

Like all visions, the problem for us is going to be how we get from where we are now to something that closely resembles the vision. From my view and the view of others general practice does seem to be reasonably well placed to develop revalidation and deliver it. The Royal College of General Practitioners (RCGP) has already rewritten *Good Medical Practice* with a GP slant.[3] We have long-established networks through the Directors of Postgraduate General Practice Education (DsPGPE), which have been developing practice and personal learning plans and other relevant professional development activities. However, we also have potential conflicts of interest developing as primary care groups, local health care co-operatives, trusts and health authorities and boards engage with governance and start to try to develop appraisal mechanisms. If these various groups do not get together and pool their resources, the end result will be confusion, chaos and a multiplicity of hoops for general practitioners to jump through, while they are being pressurised to deliver ever more and better services.

So what are the problem areas that we as a profession need to tackle if revalidation is to be developed and implemented in general practice within the timescale that has been proposed? One way of looking at these areas is to focus on systems, processes, education, resources and rigour.

Systems

Revalidation will have to be underpinned by some type of administrative system. Someone in each region is going to have to set up a system that will track general practitioners' progress through the revalidation process, and ensure that appraisals take place, that evidence is submitted on time and that revalidation groups are selected and meet. This will require development work, administrative skills and some basics such as an office and technology support. It is not yet clear who will do this. It could be the trusts, it could be the primary care groups or equivalents, it might be the RCGP or it might be the DsPGPE. What is more important is that we do not yet know how we shall achieve consensus on whose responsibility it should be.

Processes

In order to deliver revalidation, the following processes will need to be developed.

- Appraisal systems are not in place in general practice, with a few exceptions. They need to be developed urgently.
- Revalidation folders need to be developed to make it easy for doctors to gather the right information with the minimum fuss. These revalidation templates need to be both paper-based and electronic.
- We need to pilot worked examples of what a revalidation folder might contain.
- We need to find a way of ensuring that doctors' time is protected so that revalidation is conducted properly.
- We need to support doctors in developing mechanisms that will track their clinical skills and help them to target their learning.
- We need cohesive and local leadership to make it all happen.
- Trusts, the RCGP, the BMA, primary care groups and their equivalent and postgraduate general practice education units all need to co-operate so that the overlaps between revalidation, governance, continuing professional development and existing initiatives and methods are as small as possible.
- We do not know who will become the local revalidation group, how they will be chosen, who will support them or how they will be convened.

Education

Revalidation cannot happen without significant investment in education and training. Appraisal does not happen on paper. It is a difficult and delicate exercise in human contact. Appraisers need to be trained, and they need to be trained well. Until we know what an appraisal system looks like, we shall not know the numbers involved. However, as there are approximately 30 000 general practitioners in the UK, even if one appraiser dealt with 10 annual appraisals that would mean training 3000 people. Some would argue that asking a general practice to appraise one colleague a month is too much anyway, so more may need to be trained.

The local revalidation groups will need training not only at the start of any process, but regularly thereafter at a national level so that the process in different regions is equitable.

All general practitioners will need an opportunity to understand how the introduction of a new system will affect them, what they are expected to do and how they will find the time to do it.

Revalidation is change management on a grand scale. We need to approach change using its existing evidence base.[4,5] However, without a sound education and dissemination system that allows everyone to raise their anxieties and concerns at an individual level, the implementation of revalidation will be difficult and may even be impossible if it is to be meaningful.

Resources

None of this can happen without resources. The size of the resource cannot be underestimated. It includes protected time to learn about revalidation, time to develop and test systems, time to carry out revalidation, and the infrastructure necessary to support leadership and administration. Where these resources are going to come from is unclear. This issue needs to be addressed urgently if revalidation is going to fledge successfully and fly properly.

Rigour

As there are no worked-up models for revalidation, it is imperative that systems are developed and rigorously tested to ensure that they do what they are meant to do, and that they are practical in the context of everyday practice. In these days of evidence-based medicine we surely cannot develop a system that does not have a rigorous research base, if it is to stand up to public scrutiny and be meaningful. One of the major problems we face is due to the timescale within which revalidation will be implemented. Rigour and tight deadlines do not go well together, and we have to try and ensure that what we do can be defended against suggestions of tokenism, genuinely protects the public and yet is practical both in terms of time and within the constraints of general practice. We have to consider questions such as whether local revalidation groups will be fair and equitable. We have to know that the suggestion that three people act as a revalidation group meets recognisable standards of reliability. We need to know whether it really is reasonable for three people to make judgements on performance, or whether we need to develop more objective criteria. We need to know whether doctors who are submitting a wide range of evidence in their folders can actually be compared against set standards (doubts have been raised about the comparability of personally constructed written evidence).[6] In many ways we are beginning to look at these issues after we have decided on the model. Having said that, we nevertheless have a responsibility both to our patients and to ourselves to make revalidation work. The alternatives are not worth contemplating.

Retraining

One of the effects of revalidation is that there will be a need for retraining of some doctors. This is going to fall into the lap of the DsPGPE, as it is difficult to see who else can support this need. This brings with it a new set of problems that can be analysed in terms of the headings listed above. This will use up an enormous amount of resource in terms of time and money, and will also need to be included in any resourcing model for revalidation.

We have only two years in which to try and solve these problems. We need to get on with it and attempt to develop pilot projects that will look at different aspects of revalidation. In my own region we have already initiated a crossover trial of two methods of revalidation. However, it will be two years before it reports, and revalidation will be in place by then, so we have to be big enough to acknowledge that what we create will only be a start and will have to be continually developed as time goes by. We are aware of other models being developed (e.g. electronic portfolios and some of the RCGP quality initiatives). However, in general there is a lack of focus on the practicalities of delivering revalidation in terms of who is really going to develop it.

My plea is that we need urgent clarity about who is responsible for what in making revalidation happen. We need to pool resources and work together. We need to sort out local leadership and responsibilities. Now is not the time for defensiveness, egotism, empire-building and power and influence games, as these would deflect us from the task in hand, and we would surely be over-taken by external influences. Now is the time for clear leadership, if we can only work out who is really going to stick their head above the parapet and be counted. The best way is probably for the organisations I mentioned earlier to sing together (hopefully in harmony) although I have a feeling that GP educators such as directors and advisers are in a strong position to bring people together locally and to start to develop local mechanisms and systems.

References

1   General Medical Council (2000) *Revalidating Doctors: Ensuring Standards, Securing the Future*. General Medical Council, London.

2   General Medical Council (1998) *Good Medical Practice*. General Medical Council, London.

3   Royal College of General Practitioners (2000) *Good Medical Practice for General Practice*. Royal College of General Practitioners, London.

4   Barnes PC (1995) Managing change. *BMJ*. **310**: 590–2.

5   Senge P (1993) *The Fifth Discipline*. Doubleday, New York.

6   Snadden D (1999) Portfolios – attempting to measure the unmeasurable? *Med Educ*. **33**: 478–9.

Workshop deliberations on revalidation

This brief report outlines the ideas and concerns generated in a workshop at the UKCRA 2000 conference designed to look briefly at revalidation and the practicalities associated with trying to deliver the GMC's vision.

The thoughts of the workshop are set out as a series of headings representing problem areas, with some possible solutions. It was recognised that revalidation is a necessity, and that we had to work with the problems and barriers to develop a model that was practical within general practice, but which was nevertheless rigorous.

Resources

The resourcing of revalidation is a constant theme. To take the heat out of the emotions it would be helpful to have some fully costed business plans, including the opportunity costs, so that the profession and the public could see the true costs. This would allow us to develop in a context of less uncertainty about the impact that revalidation will have on clinical time. The clinical service is already stretched, so revalidation cannot be seen as an 'add-on' to the existing workload if it is to be meaningful.

Overvisiting

There is a real concern that efforts to integrate revalidation with trust initiatives associated with clinical governance have not yet started. There is a need for national co-ordination of various visiting processes in order to minimise the impact on clinical time. It is not clear who would be responsible for this national co-ordination.

Appraisal

There is considerable confusion over the definition of appraisal. Appraisal can be educational, motivational or performance-related. Each of these has different connotations for different people. We rapidly need to define what we mean by appraisal, so that we can begin to develop sensible models. One suggestion is that we work on a model which combines the elements mentioned above that produces an annual learning plan based on practitioner need. Any appraisal method will need serious investment in training.

There is also a need to ensure that the confusion which currently exists over whether revalidation is about detecting poor performance or about enhancing individual development is clarified. There are some concerns that revalidation is trying to be both, but that the two functions might be mutually exclusive.

Who makes the judgements?

There was concern that judgements relating to revalidation will need to be well thought through. The GP educators (directors and advisers) are in a strong position to assist the development of the processes both locally and nationally, as they have been involved in the design and delivery of educational quality systems for some time. In addition, they may be key facilitators in bringing local groups together to create a sense of direction in the development of revalidation.

Evidence

There is recognition that the research base underpinning revalidation is weak. However, this should be seen as a spur to develop that research base, rather than as a reason for avoiding revalidation. The systems need to be developed and implemented, and then refined as the research base strengthens.

Leadership

There are several bodies that need to be involved in the leadership of revalidation for general practice at a national level. The workshop felt that at present the leadership is unclear. The workshop identified the key stakeholders as the Committee of GP Education Directors (COGPED), the Royal College of General Practitioners (RCGP), the General Practice Committee (GPC), the primary care trusts, patients and the General Medical Council (GMC). One suggestion was that a Royal Commission on revalidation, or a similar body, could be created to bring these groups together to provide a national vision and allow strong and clear leadership to emerge. The beginnings of such a group might rest within the revalidation working group, but as yet this does not have much of a national profile.

Publicity

General practice has already done much to prepare for revalidation. *Good Medical Practice* has been rewritten for GPs, the RCGP has developed a number of quality initiatives, and the directors have a robust network of educators and expertise. We need a good publicity machine to help disseminate to the nation both what we have done and what we are going to do to improve patient care and ensure that revalidation works.

41

A view from the BMA General Practitioners' Committee

Laurence Buckman

The General Practitioners' Committee (GPC) believes that revalidation should be an educational exercise without threat for the vast majority of GPs. Opportunities for growth should take precedence over the potential to punish those who need help. We have been very disappointed by the proposals of the English Chief Medical Officer, who is committed to the punishment of GPs and the use of threat and management intervention. The General Medical Council has adopted a consultant/employee model that GPs will find difficult to work with. The GPC and the Royal College of General Practitioners are negotiating with the GMC to alter their plans to make them more appropriate for GPs.

Part 11

A health service of all the talents: the future of workforce development in the NHS

One million people work for the NHS, and £2 billion are spent on supporting the education and training of clinical staff in the NHS. However, there have been long-standing concerns about the way in which the NHS educates, trains and uses its staff to deliver the best healthcare possible for patients.[1] The government has signalled its intentions by engaging in a national consultation exercise that will eventually lead to a radical shake-up of the education, training and work-force planning systems within the NHS in England, and similar reviews have been launched in Scotland and Wales.

In this final part of the GP jigsaw, Nicholas Greenfield, the dynamic director of the Birmingham and Solihull Education Consortium, points out some of the proposed changes that will have a major effect on all of us working in the NHS.

References

1   Department of Health (2000) *A Health Service of All the Talents: Developing the NHS Work-force. A Consultation Document on the Review of Work-force Planning, April 2000.* Department of Health, London.

42

Wither education consortia: welcome confederations?

Nicholas Greenfield

In April 2000, the Department of Health published a national review of work-force development in the NHS entitled *A Health Service of All the Talents.*[1] A health authority chief executive and the deputy director of human resources at the NHS Executive wrote the review. It was based on extensive interviews throughout the NHS and captured many wide-ranging concerns about work-force planning, staffing and staff development. The main findings of the review fell within the following three main areas:

1   the NHS interface with education providers
2   changes required to the medical work-force
3   weaknesses in the management of work-force development.

The NHS interface with education providers

The review confirmed that most clinical education was undertaken on a uniprofessional basis, that there had been a significant recent increase in emphasis on academic study, and that those teaching clinical skills had often not practised them for many years. As a result, NHS managers were increasingly concerned about the fitness for its purpose of current training and the preparation of individuals to work effectively as members of multidisciplinary teams. The review therefore proposed more joint appointments between the NHS and education providers, and stressed the need to encourage more flexible, multiprofessional education.

Changes required to the medical work-force

Not surprisingly, the review identified that there were too few doctors in England and Wales, with particular recruitment problems for specialist registrars (SpRs) in some of the less popular specialities. Concern was also expressed that increasing service pressure forced Senior House Officers (SHOs) to devote a disproportionate amount of their time to service delivery rather than to education. Moreover, there was a growing tendency among SHOs to specialise at an early stage of their careers in the hope that this might improve their chances of securing the SpR post of their choice. The review suggested that this was undesirable, and it proposed the restoration of the SHO as a broad training grade. It reinforced the need to conclude negotiations about consultant work practices, contracts and job plans, which together with the development of new forms of worker (e.g. surgeon's assistant) would help to relieve service pressure on junior doctors. It also suggested the introduction of improved careers advice and professional development for all doctors – especially non-career consultant grades, who were perceived to be most neglected under the current arrangements.

Weaknesses in the management of work-force development

Perhaps the most extensive problems identified in the review concerned the management of work-force development. In particular, undergraduate medical education, postgraduate medical education and non-medical education were funded separately and often managed by different individuals or organisations. There was therefore little consistency with regard to what was funded, and insufficient co-ordination in work-force planning and the development of education infrastructure. More importantly, health authorities were inadequately engaged in these processes and work-force planning was rarely properly integrated with service or financial planning.

Responses to the review

The Department of Health received over 400 responses during the consultation period of the review. Several of these highlighted the fact that the report was biased towards secondary healthcare and failed to take proper account of primary care or dentistry. Nevertheless, there was general support for the introduction of a more integrated, holistic approach to work-force development that included all staff and placed service needs ahead of traditional professional boundaries.

The way ahead

Ministers have agreed in principle that the management and funding of education within the NHS should be reorganised. The 40 geographically based education consortia which currently manage non-medical education and training will be replaced in April 2001 by approximately 20 larger, better resourced new organisations called education confederations.

Confederations will begin with a limited set of functions, but their role will expand over two or three years to include the following functions for all staff within their local health economy:

- integrated work-force planning to deliver local health improvement programmes
- commissioning and managing education and training for all clinical staff
- working with education providers (including medical schools) to ensure sufficient high-quality placements
- managing a streamlined allocation of resources for education and training
- encouraging consistency in human resource policy and practice among constituent members, including agreed supra-employer issues such as recruitment and retention, accommodation for trainees and continuous professional development
- co-ordinating the strategic management of local learning and education facilities (e.g. education centres, libraries and skills laboratories)
- establishing robust working relationships with Learning and Skills Councils, University for Industry, Basic Skills Agency, and the NHS's own learning infrastructure.

Advantages of the new system

It is not yet clear how existing deaneries or general practice education will fit within the confederation framework. However, I hope that most people will view the change as an opportunity rather than a threat. For example, the creation of a single income stream for all education and development will enable much quicker and easier investment in educational facilities or additional staff to support libraries, information systems and clinical placements in both primary and secondary care. Better still, such investment will be strategically driven to meet the identified education priorities required to support the local health improvement programme.

Hopefully, each confederation will also have significant delegated financial authority. This could be used, for example, to ensure that GPs were equitably rewarded for training not only undergraduate medical students, but also PRHOs and other clinicians. In time it might also be sensible to put all education funding within the same income stream, rather than leaving some in trust baselines and others in GMS budgets. In this way, any increase in education required as a result of a new initiative (e.g. clinical governance) would stand a better chance of attracting additional funding.

The new arrangements should also promote opportunities for multidisciplinary education and enhance the quality of patient care. Protected time could be introduced for practice nurses to attend appropriate elements of GP registrar training. New roles, such as healthcare support workers in primary care, could be developed to release practice nurses to undertake more complex tasks, or to increase their time available for patient consultation.

If there is a danger in the new arrangements, it is that the new confederations may be so large that they cannot retain the active engagement and strong sense of ownership that a smaller, local organisation might enjoy. However, this is not unlike the problem that faces primary care groups (PCGs) as they move to primary care trust (PCT) status. Experience within consortia has shown that those PCGs which make the effort to participate in their local consortium normally improve their access to scarce resources and organisational development skills. The opportunities for working closely with confederations are likely to be even greater.

The message is clear. Wither consortia – welcome confederations!

References

1   Department of Health (2000) *A Health Service of All the Talents: Developing the NHS Work-force. A Consultation Document on the Review of Work-force Planning, April 2000*. Department of Health, London.

Index